Interferential Therapy

Interferential Therapy

by
Brenda Savage MSc, MCSP, DipTP

with contributions from
A. G. McC. Deller MSc, CEng, MBES *and*
J. R. Roberts BSc, PhD, CEng, MIERE, MBES

Wolfe Publishing Ltd

Published by
Wolfe Publishing Ltd
Brook House
2–16 Torrington Place
London WC1E 7LT

Reprinted 1992, by Richard Clay Ltd, Bungay, Suffolk

First published in 1984 by Faber and Faber Limited. Reprinted
1990.

ISBN 0 7234 1831 4

For full details of all Wolfe titles please write to Wolfe Publishing
Ltd, Brook House, 2–16 Torrington Place, London WC1E 7LT,
England.

British Library Cataloging in Publication Data

Savage, Brenda
Interferential therapy
I. Electrotherapeutics
I. Title
615.8'45   RM871

ISBN 0 7234 1831 4

Contents

List of Illustrations

Author's Preface

Having used interferential therapy since it was first introduced into the United Kingdom, I have been asked frequently to produce some kind of 'guide book' for those physiotherapists using the current for the first time. Being convinced of the current's efficacy in many, but certainly not all, conditions, I have tried, in this short book, to indicate those methods which I have found most helpful over the years.

In the early days all the literature was in foreign journals and not available. Many treatments were therefore largely empirical and I have indicated the lines of thought by which my treatment methods have been devised. These are not the only methods, and this book cannot be said to be a definitive text: it is essentially an attempt to help physiotherapists to understand how the current works and how to devise suitable and effective treatment for a number of conditions.

I am appreciative of the contributions from Mr Alastair G. McC. Deller MSc, CEng, MBES, Senior Electronics Engineer, Department of Medical Electronics, St Bartholomew's Hospital, London and Dr John R. Roberts BSc, PhD, CEng, MIERE, MBES, Director, Wolfson Centre for Medical Electronics, St Bartholomew's Hospital, London. They have described succinctly the physics of the current as well as providing excellent advice concerning the checking and testing of the machines used. I am most grateful to them.

Mrs E. M. Oakley MCSP has been painstaking in reading the original script and has been extremely generous in offering constructive suggestions. I acknowledge her help with thanks. Thanks also to Mr C. Reddihough for taking the photographs and to Mrs A. Besterman for the line drawings.

Some references and indications for further reading have been included, but such sources are limited. Readers who wish to seek further information may find that medical libraries can consult computer lists to produce the more erudite references.

Glossary

after-pain   A pain suffered by a patient some time after treatment has finished, usually due to over-dosage

capacitance   The property that allows a system or body to store an electric charge

capacitor (condenser)   A component of a circuit which stores electric charge thus offering high impedance to a low frequency current and a low impedance to a high frequency current

hertz (Hz)   The unit of frequency. In the United Kingdom sometimes expressed as cycle per second

impedance   The resistance to flow of alternating current (AC) by capacitors and coils, which varies with the frequency of the current

nociceptive nervous system   The network of nerve fibres separate from, but connected to, the central nervous system, which is responsible for the appreciation of pain

trigger point   A point distant from a lesion where the patient feels pain. Treatment which is directed at this point influences the circulation at the site of the lesion because of the autonomic connection

1. Physical Principles of Interferential Therapy

by A. G. McC. Deller MSc, CEng, MBES

HISTORICAL BACKGROUND

The concept of interferential therapy was first introduced by Dr Nemec in Vienna in the early 1950s and was practised by a few physiotherapists in Great Britain soon afterwards. The introduction of this technique, however, coincided with the arrival of powerful new drugs such as cortisone and phenylbutazone (Butazolidin) and this, combined with the fact that electrotherapy was mainly considered to be a palliative form of treatment at that time, led to its virtual disappearance.

During the late 1960s and 1970s, many of these drugs, though effective, were found to have limitations and some showed unwanted side-effects. At the same time, work on pain mechanisms by Melzak, Wall and others led to the discovery that pain could be relieved by stimulating primary afferent neurones. These and other factors have given rise to a resurgence of interest in interferential therapy, and the technique is now in general use in this country.

THE THERAPEUTIC EFFECTS OF ELECTRICAL ENERGY

The therapeutic effects of electrical energy have occupied an important position in physical medicine for many years, and a wide range of frequencies from direct current (DC) to radio and even microwave frequencies have been used.

The two principal therapeutic effects of electrical energy are the generation of heat and the stimulation of excitable tissue. The passage of electric current of any frequency through the body will give rise to the dissipation of heat, the heat generated being the product of the square of the current and the resistance of the tissue through which it flows. The stimulation of excitable tissue, on the other hand, is only possible at relatively low frequencies and those up to about 150Hz are generally used.

Where a heating effect only is required, very high frequencies are used. A typical example of this is short wave diathermy equipment which emits electrical energy at about 27MHz and is used to raise the temperature of the part of the body to be treated by approximately two degrees centigrade (2°C). The first reason for this choice of frequency is that it is too high to cause any stimulation. The second reason relates to the problem of transferring the energy from the generator to the treatment site. The skin and tissue layers may be considered electrically as capacitors. The impedance of a capacitor decreases as the frequency increases and, at short wave diathermy frequencies, the impedance of the capacitor formed by the outer layers of skin is very small and the vast majority of the energy supplied by the generator will be dissipated in the bulk of the tissue. A further important advantage of using this high frequency is that the energy may be capacitively coupled to the body without there being any direct contact between electrodes and skin.

When excitable tissue functions, cell membranes undergo transient alterations in permeability and allow the rapid passage of ions across them. This flow of ions constitutes an electric current which, flowing through resistive tissue, gives rise to an electric field on the surface of the body. These changing fields therefore reflect the activity of excitable tissue and are often recorded and used diagnostically, as in the case of the electrocardiogram.

Like many other biological processes, this is reversible. The application of an external electric field can cause ionic currents to flow in excitable tissue.

In the resting state, there normally exists a potential difference of approximately 0.1 volts across a neural membrane. If this potential is reversed for at least 20 microseconds, the neurone will be stimulated and an action potential propagated.

Different types of excitable tissue propagate impulses at widely differing speeds. This fact, combined with differing stimulus duration requirements shown by strength-duration curves, means that for each type of excitable tissue there is an optimum frequency at which the maximum response will be elicited. Some typical examples are quoted below:

0–5Hz	sympathetic nerves
10–150Hz	parasympathetic nerves
10–50Hz	motor nerves
90–110Hz	sensory nerves
130Hz	nociceptive system
0–10Hz	unstriped muscle

There are a number of problems that arise in trying to treat the body at these frequencies, particularly in the case of deep seated lesions. The low frequency currents may well not only stimulate the target tissue, but also other tissues through which they pass. The dry outer corneal layer of the skin is of relatively high resistance and the capacitance between these layers mentioned previously will contribute little to reducing the overall impedance at these frequencies. Another problem when applying DC or very low frequencies is that of electrolysis of fluid in the tissues causing ulceration at the sites of application. It is primarily these considerations that have led to the development of interferential therapy.

THE THEORY OF INTERFERENTIAL THERAPY

In interferential therapy, two medium frequency alternating currents of slightly differing frequencies are applied to the body in such a way that they cross and interact to produce a low frequency therapeutic current at the relevant point.

When two currents of differing frequencies are allowed to interact, an interesting effect occurs. Consider the two currents A and B shown in Figure 1/1. Current A is a sine wave of frequency f_1 and current B is also a sine wave of the same amplitude as A but of slightly higher frequency, f_2. When the two are added together, the current waveform C will result. It

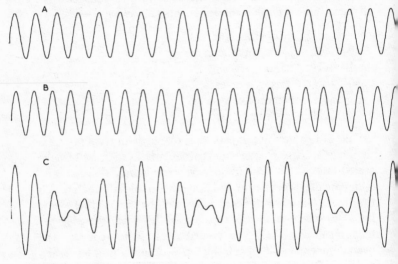

Fig. 1/1   The phenomenon of beating

will be observed that current B falls alternately into and out of step with current A, alternately reinforcing and weakening it. This resultant waveform is also sinusoidal having a frequency $\tilde{f}$, where $\tilde{f}$ is a frequency between f_1 and f_2. In the special case where the amplitudes of A and B are exactly equal, $\tilde{f}$ will be the mean of A and B, i.e. $\tilde{f} = (f_1 + f_2)/2$.

The amplitude of this waveform, however, is not constant – it varies sinusoidally with a frequency $f_2 - f_1$. This phenomenon is known as beating, $f_2 - f_1$ is the beat frequency resulting from the addition of A and B. The current C, a sine wave of frequency $\bar{f}$, is said to be amplitude modulated by f_2–f_1. Amplitude modulation is widely used in radio communications. It is important to note that the current C consists of a single frequency, $\bar{f}$, in order to extract the low frequency it must first be demodulated. Demodulation may be achieved by introducing a non-linearity into the system and in radio communications the non-linear characteristic of a diode is often used. In the case of interferential therapy, it is fortunate that cell membranes exhibit non-linear characteristics as these enable endogenous demodulation of the interference current, extracting the low frequency therapeutic current at the site of interference.

In interferential therapy machines, the medium frequency currents applied to the body are normally at a frequency of about 4000Hz, this being a frequency at which the effective skin impedance is at a minimum. Employing the nomenclature used above, a typical interferential therapy machine would give outputs as follows – frequency A would be fixed at 4000Hz and frequency B would be variable from 4010Hz to 4150Hz. This would give a choice of therapeutic frequencies, i.e. f_2–f_1, from 10Hz to 150Hz.

The foregoing explanation has assumed two currents of equal magnitude flowing in a homogeneous medium; in practice, this is unlikely. The body is not homogeneous from an electrical point of view, the electrical properties of muscle, bone and fat are all different and therefore the distribution of the electric field will not be completely even. This, combined with the fact that exactly symmetrical placing of all four electrodes with respect to the treatment site is rarely possible due to the limitations imposed by the external body contours, means that the impedance presented to each of the two pairs of electrodes is unlikely to be equal. Some interferential therapy machines, therefore, provide a balance control enabling the output of one channel to be increased while the other is decreased, thus allowing the operator to balance the intensities of the two currents.

The situation obtaining when the two currents are not equal is shown in Figure 1/2. Beating will still occur, but its amplitude will be less and will be superimposed on a common beating amplitude. The situation shown in Figure 1/1 is referred to as full beating or 100 per cent modulation. In the case of Figure 1/2 we have partial beating or less than 100 per cent modulation. The percentage modulation is known as the depth of modulation.

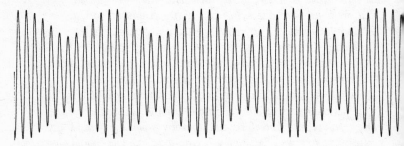

Fig. 1/2   Partial beating

THE SPATIAL DISTRIBUTION OF INTERFERENTIAL CURRENTS

Physical quantities such as mass and length may be completely defined in terms of magnitude only, these are referred to as scalar quantities. In order to completely define a current of a particular frequency at a point in an interference field, however, information as to both its magnitude and direction must be provided. Such quantities are termed *vector* quantities. These quantities may be represented diagramatically by a line called a vector. The magnitude of the vector is represented by its length and its direction by the angle measured between it and a reference direction.

In Figures 1/1 and 1/2 it has been assumed that the two

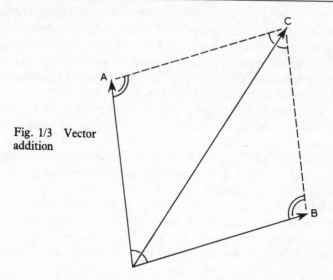

Fig. 1/3 Vector addition

currents A and B are flowing in the same direction. In practice, of course, the directions of A and B will be approximately at right angles to one another. The effect of this is shown vectorially in Figure 1/3, current C being the vector sum of currents A and B. All the frequencies will be the same as in the first example, but the magnitude and direction of the resultant current, C, will be different.

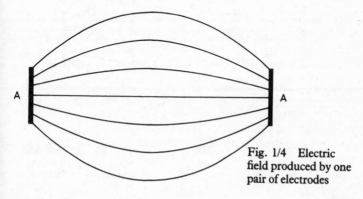

Fig. 1/4 Electric field produced by one pair of electrodes

The passage of current through a pair of electrodes applied to a medium will result in the creation of a field throughout that medium as shown in Figure 1/4. The lines of force represent the directions of maximum intensity and the maximum intensity of the current at any point within the medium can be represented by a vector tangential to the line of force at that point.

It is important to note at this juncture that, while the vectors shown in Figure 1/4 represent the directions of maximum intensity, components of this current will exist in all directions, albeit of reduced magnitude. If the application of a second field is now considered, as in the case of interferential therapy, the result will be as shown in Figure 1/5. At any point, x, within the medium there will be two directions in which the component due to current A and that due to B will be equal, and therefore full beating will occur in those directions although the amplitude of the beating may be different in each case. In the

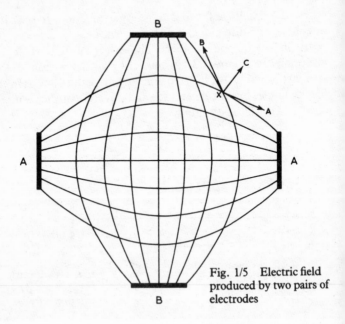

Fig. 1/5   Electric field produced by two pairs of electrodes

direction at right angles to A, the component due to A will obviously be zero and at right angles to B the component due to B will be zero. This means that, in these two directions, no beating will occur. In summary, at all points in the medium there will be two directions in which full beating will occur and two in which none will occur. In all other directions, some beating will occur.

The impression is sometimes given that the interference field produced by interferential therapy machines comprises a number of single, narrow vectors. The previous discussion shows that this is clearly not the case. The interference currents are the result of the interaction of two electric fields, both of which pervade the entire medium. Interference currents will thus occur at all points in the medium and in all directions, although they will, of course, vary widely in magnitude.

Many interferential therapy machines are provided with one or two current meters on the front panel. It is important to realise that these meters only indicate the magnitude of the medium frequency currents that the machine is supplying to the patient, they do not show the magnitude of any low frequency therapeutic currents that may be produced.

FREQUENCY SWING

The above discussion has assumed that the two applied frequencies are constant, producing a constant therapeutic beat frequency. A constant beat frequency, though widely used, has two principal disadvantages. Firstly, it may be desired to treat several types of excitable tissue during one treatment, each with differing optimum frequencies of excitation. Secondly, there is the problem of accommodation or the habituation response. In this case, the response of a particular type of excitable tissue decreases with time as the tissue accommodates to the stimulating frequency.

This problem is overcome in many interferential therapy

machines by the provision of a facility for *frequency swing*, sometimes referred to as spectrum or *sweep*. Machines, as already explained, provide two medium frequency outputs, one fixed and one variable. When frequency swing is required, the machine will automatically swing the variable frequency output between specified limits, resulting in a varying beat frequency. The precise way in which the operator sets the frequencies varies from machine to machine. In some cases it is only possible to select a fixed range of swing about the desired therapeutic beat frequency, other machines permit the setting of the upper and lower limits of swing thus allowing the operator to choose any range of swing.

Several types of swing pattern may also be provided. One swing pattern simply switches from one frequency to another, e.g. six seconds at the lower frequency followed by six seconds at the higher frequency. The time between switching may also be variable. Another swing pattern commonly used is a variable sweep, the output will gradually increase over a period of, say, six seconds from the the lower to the higher frequency and then decrease to the lower frequency in a further six seconds. The swing facilities provided on different machines vary considerably and it is important that the operator understands those provided on the particular machine in use.

Small sweeps of 10Hz or so are often used to overcome the problem of accommodation. Wider sweeps will enable a greater range of excitable tissue to be stimulated, but it is important to remember that the wider the swing the less will be the time that a particular type of excitable tissue will be receiving its optimum frequency.

OTHER TREATMENT MODES

Bipolar mode

In this case, only two electrodes are applied to the patient and the two medium frequency currents are added inside the machine to produce an output similar to current C in Figure 1/1. Endogenous demodulation of this amplitude modulated current will take place and a low frequency therapeutic current will be produced. This current will, however, be distributed in the same way as conventional stimulating currents. This treatment mode is sometimes referred to as 'electrokinesy'.

Diadynamic therapy

This treatment mode also uses a medium frequency amplitude modulated current and is also applied using two electrodes only. In this case, however, the waveform is half-wave rectified, producing amplitude modulated DC impulses.

'Rotating vector' systems

These systems attempt to extend the effectiveness of conventional interferential therapy by causing the essentially static interference field to change direction in a rhythmical manner. This is achieved by varying the two outputs of the machine sinusoidally and in phase opposition at very low frequencies.

Stereodynamic systems

In this case, three pairs of electrodes are used and the machine provides three outputs. The advantages claimed for this system being that it produces a more three-dimensional field with beat frequencies of increased complexity, thus improving the spread of the low frequency therapeutic currents and decreasing accommodation problems.

SELECTED REFERENCES

De Domenico, G. (1981). *Basic Guidelines for Interferential Therapy*. Theramed Books, Sydney, Australia.

Ganne, J. M. (1976). Interferential therapy. *Australian Journal of Physiotherapy*, **22**, 3, 101–10.

Hansjurgens, A. (1975). Dynamic interference current therapy. *Physikslische Medizin und Rehabilitation*, **311**, 1.

Richards, J. P. G. and Williams, R. P. (1972). *Waves*. Penguin Library of Physical Sciences: Physics. Penguin Books, Harmondsworth.

ACKNOWLEDGEMENT

The author thanks Dr R. J. Treffene of Queensland Institute of Technology, Brisbane, Australia for his valuable work on theoretical models of interferential fields.

See also page 34.

2. Practical Considerations in Interferential Therapy

by J. R. Roberts BSc, PhD, CEng, MIERE, MBES

It is important to realise that some therapeutic electrical stimulators such as those found in interferential therapy machines are capable of generating large (strong) electric currents. If applied incorrectly these currents can cause discomfort to the patient and in exceptional circumstances may be potentially hazardous.

Initially, the physiotherapist has to assume that the safety and well-being of the patient is assured when the particular instrument is working correctly and used in accordance with its operating instructions. This relies on the equipment manufacturer employing good design and manufacturing techniques and abiding by the current national standards applying to that type of equipment.

Recently, the electrical safety standards controlling the design and construction of electro-medical equipment have been strengthened by the introduction of a new standard. This standard exists in two largely identical forms; as an International Standard IEC 601–1 and as an equivalent British Standard, BS 5724 part 1 (see p. 30). While a detailed discussion of these standards is completely beyond the scope of this chapter, there are a number of basic points which are discussed here since appreciation of them will assist the therapist when using electrical physiotherapy apparatus.

It is important to know how to identify those units claiming compliance with BS 5724. This information is contained in characteristic identifying marks normally placed on the rear panel of the instrument.

It is also very important, and now compulsory within the National Health Service (NHS), that those medical authorities purchasing electro-medical equipment should ensure that it complies with BS 5724. Outside the United Kingdom (UK) the situation is confused although most European countries recognise IEC 601–1 or have their own version of it.

These standards are designed to protect both the patient and therapist from the hazards of inadequate electrical equipment and include in their specifications some aspects of the following:

Mechanical (physical) design and construction

Under this heading the strength of panels, the size and type of fixing screw on access covers and the method of securing the mains lead are specified.

Labelling of controls and general marking

The controls on an instrument must be clearly marked if it is to be used correctly and there are clauses in the standards which cover the design and legibility as well as the resistance to abrasion of the marks on the front and rear panels of the equipment. Apart from this, there are several special types which may be encountered by physiotherapists.

The mains switch on the instrument may be labelled 'On' and 'Off' although these same functions may also be represented by a '1' and a '0' respectively (presumably to overcome any language barrier).

It is obviously good practice for an operator to read the instruction manual before using a piece of equipment for the first time. For this purpose the symbol shown in Figure 2/1 has been introduced. It may be seen on the front panel of physiotherapy machines and carries the official definition:

Attention – Consult Accompanying Documents

There are other symbols which relate directly to the electrical

Fig. 2/1 Specialised symbols BS 5724: (a) Caution; (b) Type B; (c) Type BF; (d) Class II

(a)   (b)   (c)   (d)

performance of the apparatus covering its general classification.

This part of the standard also includes the marking of the fuses to allow their correct replacement which is extremely important if the equipment is not to overheat when a fault occurs.

Electrical performance

One of the concepts behind all electrical safety standards is the need for the particular apparatus to remain in a safe state even in the presence of a fault condition. Many physiotherapy machines are powered from the mains supply and housed in a metal enclosure, which will generally be earthed via the mains lead. Apart from acting as a container for the internal parts the enclosure also prevents the operator or the patient contacting any of the high and possibly hazardous voltages within it. As a result of the small capacitance (stray capacitance) between the metal case and those components inside it which are connected to the mains supply there is a small *leakage current* which flows from the instrument enclosure to earth. The maximum value of this current is specified by the standard and although not hazardous it is preferable that it does not flow through either the patient or operator under fault conditions.

The equipment described in the previous paragraph with an earthed metal housing is described as being *Class 1*. Where such an instrument acts as an electrical stimulator it is possible that one of the patient electrodes is also earthed. This condition is shown diagrammatically in Figure 2/2a and the apparatus is described as *Class 1 Type B*. It should be apparent by looking at the diagram that if the earth connection at the wall socket is interrupted the leakage current will try to flow through the patient. Often, as with interferential therapy machines which

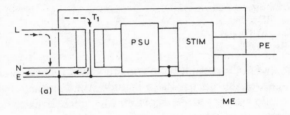

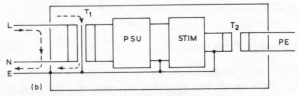

Fig. 2/2   Schematic representation of equipment
classification: (a) Class 1 Type B; (b) Class 1 Type BF. *Key*:
L=line; N=neutral; E=earth (mains supply); T_1=mains
transformer; T_2=output transformer; PSU=power supply
unit; STIM=stimulator electronics; ME=metal instrument
enclosure; - - →=leakage current path; PE=patient electrodes

supply alternating current output it is possible for the internal
stimulator circuits to be connected to the patient electrodes via a
transformer. This isolating transformer acts as a further
safeguard making it more difficult for the fault currents,
mentioned previously, to flow into the patient. Such equipment
is often described as having a 'floating' patient circuit and is
described by the standards as being *Class 1 Type BF* (Fig. 2/2b).

Equipment complying with IEC 601–1 or BS 5724 pt 1
must carry a label listing the Class and Type, and an interferential therapy machine could be marked on the rear panel:
BS 5724 pt 1 Class 1 Type BF.

As well as carrying these labels the panel of the instrument
may also include one of the two pictorial representations shown
in Figure 2/1. Here the 'stick figure' symbolises Class 1 Type B,
while the boxed figure is Class 1 Type BF.

A further symbol that may be encountered on the back of a

physiotherapy machine is Figure 2/1d. This symbol, the double square, represents equipment in Class II. Unlike Class 1, instruments in this category are unearthed and will invariably be housed in a plastics case and may also be battery powered. Domestic examples of this class are some electric power equipment such as drills and lawn mowers, and examination of their power cords will reveal that the green/yellow earth conductor is missing. Class II physiotherapy equipment is specially constructed, using double insulation, which provides an extra layer of electrical safety and this makes the third conductor superfluous.

USE OF ELECTRICAL/ELECTRONIC EQUIPMENT

Unfortunately BS 5724 can do little to control how the equipment is used or abused. It is inevitable that from time to time equipment will fail to operate properly especially if it is used frequently by different operators. There are a number of simple precautions and checks that the physiotherapist can employ to minimise problems and ensure that the interferential equipment is working correctly.

Controls

It is essential that the physiotherapist is completely familiar with the operating controls of the equipment before treating a patient. Interferential therapy machines will normally include some form of cut-out to prevent the current(s) being applied to the patient inadvertently when the machine is first switched on.

This is a very valuable safety feature which can cause some problems if misunderstood. The cut-out is reset by reducing the output level control to the minimum position at which time the cut-out indication, often a lamp, should go off.

Confusion can arise when using machines that have the

facility to control the output remotely. Where there is a local/remote switch on the front panel it is likely that selecting the remote position without the remote control plugged in will put the cut-out on as a precaution. Setting the output to the minimum setting will not reset the cut-out until either the remote control is plugged in or the local position selected on the front panel.

Leads

It is important that the leads are in good condition otherwise the therapeutic equipment may not operate reliably. Each flexible lead consists of several strands of very fine copper wire laid together to form a single conductor. This conductor is contained within a PVC insulating jacket.

MAINS LEAD

Frequently two or more of these wires are grouped inside an outer sheath to form a composite cable. In the case of a mains lead each of the three conductors normally consists of 24 strands of copper wire 0.2mm in diameter. Where the mains lead enters the instrument via a mains connector it is possible for the operation of the machine to be intermittent if this connector is not pushed well in. This may easily happen if the equipment is mounted on a trolley and the lead is left trailing on the floor when not in use.

PATIENT LEAD

If the patient lead is not reliable by being damaged or worn the electrical circuit, i.e. connection, between the machine and the patient may be intermittent. It may be connected and disconnected at random when the patient or the lead is moved slightly. This will certainly cause the current flowing through the electrodes to surge in a very uncomfortable way. The exact perception of this by the patient will vary, depending on the patient as well as the particular output level. However, the patient will be startled and may report that they felt an electric shock.

Electrodes

It is very important for the comfort and protection of the patient that the electrodes are in good condition and are correctly applied. There is a wide variety of electrode styles in use in electrotherapy – the two most common ones being plate and suction cup electrodes (see Chapter 3).

Since the leads and electrodes on any piece of electrotherapy equipment receive considerable wear if they are in frequent use it is very important that from time to time the physiotherapist checks that these components are functioning correctly.

Simple checks

After turning on the interferential therapy machine the physiotherapist can check that the instrument, leads and electrodes are all working correctly in the following way.

Make sure that the electrodes, their leads and the patient lead, are connected both together and into the output socket on the interferential therapy machine. Connect each pair of electrodes together to form a short circuit retaining them with a clip or weight. After selecting the four-electrode method the output control can be turned up to see if full output can be obtained on both channels. If this is not possible on either channel then that channel may be at fault. If moving the patient lead or electrode lead causes the output indicator (meter) to fluctuate significantly this indicates that an intermittent connection is likely. It may be possible to locate the broken/loose connection more closely by moving individual parts of the leads; the faulty item can then be replaced. If it is the wires in the electrode lead that are broken this may be recognised by checking if the lead is elastic and stretches at some point.

If a vacuum unit is in use a similar procedure can be followed.

First link this unit to the interferential unit, then by folding the cups inside out and pressing the plates together (using a bulldog or other paper clip) the circuits can be tested as before.

Short wave interference

Unfortunately, the strong electric fields generated by the use of a short wave diathermy machine can have a very disruptive effect on the lower power electronic circuits contained in an electrical stimulator like an interferential therapy unit. If it is necessary to use the two in close proximity to one another, e.g. in adjacent cubicles, a check should be made to make sure that the interferential unit contains a filter circuit to minimise the short wave interference. The manufacturer's handbook should contain this information together with the recommended minimum distance between the two when both are in use. In spite of this it is a wise precaution with new equipment for the therapist to check the operation of the machine either with the electrodes clamped together (or carefully on a volunteer) before treating a patient when a short wave unit is in use nearby.

REFERENCES

IEC 601–1 *Safety of Medical Electrical Equipment*, part 1: *General Requirements*. International Electrotechnical Commission.

BS 5724: Part 1: 1979 *Safety of Medical Electrical Equipment: General Requirements*. British Standards Institution, London.

ACKNOWLEDGEMENT

John Roberts and Alastair Deller wish to acknowledge the Director and staff of the Department of Medical Electronics, St Bartholomew's Hospital, London for supporting the work on which these two opening chapters are based.

CHECK LIST FOR INTERFERENTIAL THERAPY EQUIPMENT

Action	Remedy
Unfamiliar machine/procedure	Check manual
Check leads and electrodes	Replace faulty items
Plug in all leads and switch on	
Check power on indicators	Check fuses/mains lead, etc; replace faulty items
Check cut-out indicator	Output to minimum (MIN) or local switch
Set up controls	
Clamp electrodes together	
Turn output to maximum	
Check output indicators for full scale	Check patient leads and electrodes
Machine ready for use	

3. Application of Interferential Therapy

TYPES OF ELECTRODES (Fig. 3/1)

Plate electrodes

The simplest type of electrode is a metal plate which should be covered with absorbent material (see below). Because metal plates are rather hard and inflexible they soon crack and become unserviceable. To overcome this manufacturers have replaced them with plates made of conducting rubber which are more comfortable, and last longer.

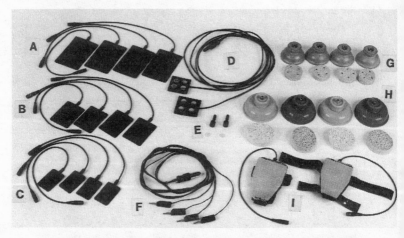

Fig. 3/1 Types of electrodes. (A) large plate electrodes; (B) medium plate electrodes; (C) small plate electrodes; (D) combined electrode; (E) combined stud electrode; (F) connection leads; (G) small vacuum electrodes; (H) large vacuum electrodes; (I) labile electrodes

The plates are of different sizes. For a *general* treatment the plates should be as large as can be accommodated on the part as this gives a more comfortable treatment and a deeper effect. If a *localised* effect is required small electrodes are used, but the effect is more superficial. It is sometimes convenient to use two large plates proximally, and two small ones distally, for example when treating the arm which is considerably larger at the deltoid than the wrist. This is quite permissible as each circuit will have one large and one small electrode so that they are still balanced. It would *not* be correct to use two small electrodes in one circuit and two large in the other.

The plates are attached to the patient by means of straps or bandages. Straps may sometimes be quicker and easier to apply, but a crêpe bandage gives a firmer and more even contact, and therefore a more comfortable treatment. While the patient will come to no actual harm if part of the electrode is not in contact, the treatment will be less pleasant and the patient will not tolerate as much current.

COVERING

The electrode covering must be absorbent. Spontex has been found to be very effective. Bags into which the different sized electrodes can be slipped are easily made. They should be soaked in water or a solution of bicarbonate of soda to improve conduction and allow a more comfortable contact with the skin.

The Spontex covers must be kept clean, and washed thoroughly and dried after use. Some departments also rinse them in a disinfectant such as Savlon. If this washing is not done effectively the covers will disintegrate producing an unpleasant odour. This is because the material supports bacteria. The thickness of the absorbent covering is immaterial as no caustic substances are produced by the alternating current. Its purpose is to ensure a comfortable and even contact. If preferred lint pads may be used instead of the Spontex.

Ordinary plastic foam does *not* conduct the current and must not be used.

Vacuum electrodes

The interferential unit is plugged into the vacuum unit. These
are really plate electrodes kept in position by a vacuum instead
of bandaging. The plate is enclosed in a rubber suction cup
connected to a machine capable of producing a vacuum, by
means of a hollow tube, through which passes an electrical
connection (Fig. 3/2). The plate lies in the back of the cup and

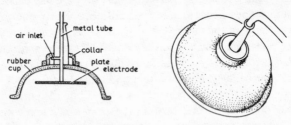

Fig. 3/2   Vacuum electrode

contact is made with the skin by means of a damp Spontex
sponge. Round the edge of the cup is a flange to allow an airtight
seal to be made with the patient's skin. The cup will adhere
more readily if this flange is damp. Round the neck of the cup is
a rubber collar covering a small hole. By lifting the collar, air is
let into the cup thus allowing the electrode to be moved while
the vacuum is in operation (should adjustment of its position be
necessary) without displacing the other electrodes. Any attempt
to tug off the electrode from the patient without releasing the
vacuum results in discomfort and bruising.

To apply the electrodes the cups are attached to the vacuum
unit taking care that the 'colour coded' tubes are connected
firmly to the correct nozzles, as otherwise the electrodes will not
be correctly identified. Firm attachment is necessary to produce
good suction. The sponges are soaked in water or a solution of
sodium bicarbonate and squeezed almost dry. If they are too wet
water would be sucked into the tubes preventing the cups from
adhering properly, or even be drawn into the vacuum unit. The

sponges are placed in the cups and the edges of the cups moistened. The vacuum unit is turned on to produce a moderate suction and the cups placed firmly on the patient in the desired position. It will be found that if the electrodes are applied in pairs they will attach more readily. If difficulty is still experienced two electrodes may be placed temporarily on the smooth surface of the apparatus where they will adhere more readily as the suction of the machine is not being dissipated. The second pair of electrodes is then placed in position on the patient. These always adhere more readily. The suction is now adjusted to be just sufficient to keep the electrodes in place. Too much suction leads to unsightly bruising, but too little allows the cups to fall off.

The suction should not be constant. It may be pulsed and adjusted to increase and decrease at a desired speed. In some vacuum units both speed and degree of suction can be varied over a whole range but push-button types give a choice of fast, medium and slow. Most patients find a rapid change irritating, and the electrodes tend to fall off. Medium frequency pulsation is usually most comfortable. Slow pulsation produces an increase in deep circulation, but may produce bruising.

A constant suction is not used as it is uncomfortable and almost always produces bruising.

Vacuum electrodes are excellent for treating flat smooth areas such as the back or a plump knee, where they can be applied quickly and easily. On bony areas such as the shoulder or ankle it is impossible to place the cup in the correct position with the whole rim in contact without deforming the cup. If the cup is squeezed as shown in Figure 3/3 the area enclosed by the rim is diminished, so the two electrodes would not be the same size

Fig. 3/3 Application of vacuum electrode: (a) right; (b) wrong. (Although the circumference is the same, the enclosed area is not)

and the circuit unbalanced. Too great suction has also to be used and, further, the cups tend to become detached if the patient moves even slightly. In such areas plate electrodes bandaged on are quicker, more comfortable and more effective. On hairy areas it is almost impossible to get an airtight seal and the cups will not stay in position. The thin papery skin of the elderly also presents difficulty with contact and bruises easily. Vacuum electrodes are unsuitable for patients who are taking steroids because of the likelihood of bruising.

Vacuum electrodes are useful for treating relatively immobile patients, such as a patient with an acute back, as they may be applied in any position in which the patient is at ease, be it standing, sitting or lying. For the patient with an arthritic hip treatment may be given in side lying; he need not be moved about either for bandaging or for changing the position of electrodes for the second part of the treatment.

In using suction cups care must be taken that the sponges are thick enough to fill the cups and make good contact. They soon become worn and thin and must be replaced. Spontex *must* be used. As previously stated plastic foam does not conduct the current and the treatment will be ineffective. This absence of current may pass unnoticed by some patients, particularly the elderly, who find it difficult to appreciate the prickling of the current when it is masked by the pulsating suction of the cups.

Combined electrodes

Combined electrodes are so constructed that all four contacts are embedded in some insulating material and can be applied as one pad. There are several sizes.

Fig. 3/4 Combined electrode: four contacts in a small cylinder

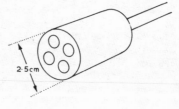

2·5 cm

In the smallest, the four contacts are enclosed in a cylinder less than 2.5cm (1in) in diameter (Fig. 3/4). Each contact is very small, so only very low intensity of current can be tolerated and the effect is very superficial. It is used to treat very localised points of pain, such as the supra-orbital nerve as it emerges from the foramen: indeed it would be difficult to treat this area using a four-electrode technique in any other way.

The medium sized electrode has the four contacts, each 1cm in diameter, embedded in a foam rubber pad (Fig. 3/5). If the contacts are bare metal they must be covered with a Spontex

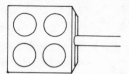

Fig. 3/5 Combined electrode: four contacts embedded in a foam rubber pad

pad; some manufacturers use material which needs no covering as it is soft enough to make contact with the skin, but difficulty may be experienced with soaking them. Little current can be used as the area of contact is so small and the effect is superficial. Such a pad is useful in treating a small area such as a single finger joint; or for giving an anaesthetising dose to a tender area, when the apparatus will not provide for a bi-polar technique (see p. 45).

The largest size has contacts about 5cm (2in) across, but otherwise is of identical construction. It has limited use, for example the treatment of the wrist or elbow in a thin patient, but unless the limb is exactly the right size the crossing point of the currents will not be accurately sited as the position of electrodes relative to each other is fixed.

Some makers produce pairs of electrodes of similar construction in the medium size. If the two pads are of equal size each represents two poles only, diagonal contacts being connected to one pole of each circuit (Fig. 3/6a). These two pads must therefore be used together to complete both circuits. They must be placed on the patient so that the leads emerge in the same

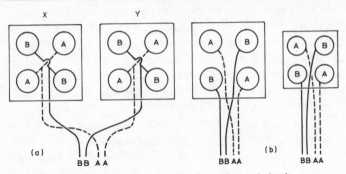

Fig. 3/6   Use of combined electrodes: (a) with equal-sized
electrodes; (b) with uneven-sized electrodes

direction; it can be seen that if (y) is rotated through 90 degrees,
there will be no crossing of the two currents and no interference.
If the two pads are of unequal size each contact is connected to a
different pole (Fig. 3/6b), so that each pad may be used
separately as the single electrode, taking care not to place the
unused pad on a conducting surface and so diverting the current
away from the patient. If used together a most complicated
interference pattern is produced, superficially under each pad
and also more deeply between the two.

Although easier to apply than four separate electrodes the use
of these electrodes is limited by the low intensity of current that
can be tolerated so the general effect is small. Ease of application
does not compensate for the relatively ineffective treatment; if it
is possible use four larger separate electrodes.

Labile electrode (Fig. 3/7)

A labile electrode is a plate electrode insulated on one side and
attached to the operator's hand by means of Velcro straps. The
conducting side is covered with Spontex, to provide contact.
Two electrodes are always used: they are held in position by the
operator and are designed to be moved over the patient's skin
during treatment.

Fig. 3/7 Labile electrode

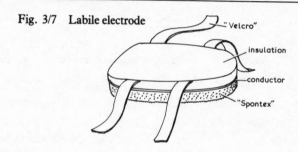

Localising electrode (Fig. 3/8)

The localising electrode is a very small plate electrode set back in a metal lined plastics cup. Contact is made by a soaked sponge filling the cup. Two such electrodes are held between the fingers of one hand to localise the current.

PLACING OF ELECTRODES

Four-electrode method (Fig. 3/9)

The classic application of interferential therapy is by the four-electrode method. For the treatment of a joint two electrodes, one from each circuit, are placed on opposite sides of the limb above the joint, and two below, so that the two currents cross within the joint. This is shown in Figure 3/10. In (a) the

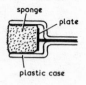

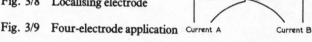

Fig. 3/8 Localising electrode

Fig. 3/9 Four-electrode application

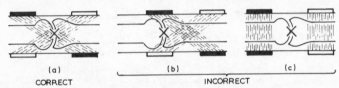

Fig. 3/10 Four-electrode application: (a) correct; (b & c) incorrect.
X=lesion

application is correctly made. In (b) although the electrodes are correctly placed for the currents to cross, they are so sited that the crossing does not occur at the site of the lesion (X). In (c) the electrodes are placed so that the currents do not cross at all and no interference occurs.

Alternatively the four electrodes may be placed on the joint, one circuit being antero-posterior and the other from side to side, to give a more localised treatment. In practice, various applications to the joint are made at subsequent attendances until the one producing the best result is found. Varying the positions of electrodes also ensures that all structures within the joint receive treatment.

Usually even-sized electrodes are used but in an uneven limb it may be convenient to use larger electrodes above the joint and smaller ones below. As one large and one small electrode is in each circuit this does not lead to imbalance.

With some apparatus it is possible, if desired, to use two vacuum electrodes and two plates. Again since one of each type is attached to each circuit there is no imbalance.

Four electrodes may also be used in a co-planar application as

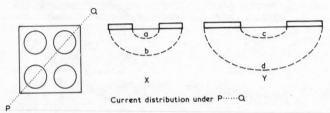

Current distribution under P·····Q

Fig. 3/11 Co-planar application to the back

in treating the back (Fig. 3/11). The depth of penetration depends on the size of the electrodes and the intensity of the current. If small electrodes are used path (a) is significantly shorter than path (b), but in (y) where large electrodes are used the spread of the current is significantly deeper before this difference is apparent. To penetrate the thickness of the back muscles without producing discomfort it is necessary to use at least the medium-sized electrodes.

Fig. 3/12 Two-electrode application:
(a) central lesion;
(b) superficial lesion;
(c) longitudinal;
(d) co-planar

(a) Centrally placed lesion

(b) Superficial lesion

(c) Longitudinal application

(d) Coplanar application

Two-electrode method (bi-polar method)

Some apparatus provides for an application using two electrodes only. The circuit is so designed that the interference is produced within the apparatus and the current, produced in one circuit only, is a low frequency modulation of the 4000Hz type. This is a similar current to that which, with the four-electrode application, is produced at the crossing point of the two currents within the body.

For this application the two electrodes are placed preferably opposite each other so that the site to be treated lies directly in the path of the current (Fig. 3/12a). If the lesion lies nearer one surface than the other, a small electrode is placed over this and a larger directing electrode on the other side of the limb

(Fig. 3/12b). This is the most accurate method of localising but when it is not anatomically possible a co-planar application is made (Fig. 3/12d). The co-planar position is also necessary if the lesion is covered by strapping or plaster, though here the four-electrode method would be preferable.

Two electrodes may also be used as a longitudinal application to treat a whole limb (Fig. 3/12c) either to increase the circulation or influence the whole length of a nerve.

The disadvantage of the bi-polar application is that there is more sensory stimulation, which many patients find unpleasant. This happens because with only one channel the amplitude of the current is varying slowly at the beat frequency. With two channels, the four-electrode method, the amplitude of each channel is constant and the low frequency current is only produced within the body and does not stimulate the skin.

On applying the two-electrode (bi-polar) *interferential* therapy, as the intensity of current is increased, the patient feels the pain reproduced or exacerbated. If he does not, the active electrode is slowly moved about until he does. It is then in the correct place and treatment may proceed. This is clearly less open to error than having to adjust four electrodes.

In practice it is found that with two patients with apparently similar conditions one will consistently respond to the four-electrode application and the other to the two-electrode method. Why this should be is not clear.

WARNING

Not all apparatus produces this particular type of interferential current. On some there is a bi-polar current called 'analgesic current' or 'impulse'. This is **not** an interferential current but is unidirectional; unless precautions are taken it can produce burns, by production of acids and alkalis under the electrodes and round any metal buried in the tissues, such as plates, screws, prostheses and sutures.

Labile method

Instead of applying two electrodes in a fixed position and giving a stable treatment they may be moved about to give a labile one. Special electrodes are used that are insulated on one side so that the current does not pass through the operator. They are attached to the hands with Velcro straps. Should these not be available an adequate treatment may be given using plate electrodes with the operator wearing rubber gloves (Fig. 3/13).

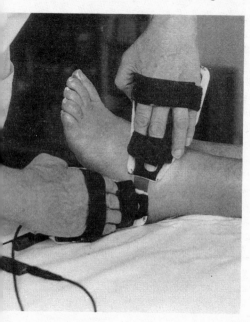

Fig. 3/13 The operator wears labile electrodes held in position with Velcro straps. She is treating a local lesion

A 100Hz current is selected. Both pads are placed on the patient and the intensity increased until a definite tingling is felt. It is helpful if a foot control is available by which the current can be increased; if it is not, both pads are held by one hand while the current is adjusted and thereafter both hands are used on the patient. The pads are then moved over the area to be treated using a see-saw movement so that the area of pad in contact with the patient alters. This varies the current density and areas of tenderness may thus be located. This surging of the current gives a very comfortable and relaxing treatment particularly for muscular conditions. Part of both pads must always be kept in contact. If one pad is lifted off entirely it is painful for the patient.

Usually both pads are moved, but in treating awkward or restricted areas such as the face, one pad is kept still and the other moved.

In treating the back or shoulder girdle with many tender points, the pads are moved over the whole area slowly. As the affected area is reached the current appears to increase. Concentrated treatment is then given to this area until it is no longer sensitive, and the pads then moved on to treat the next area. On returning to the area later in the treatment it will be found that the increased sensitivity has gone.

In the old apparatus this labile treatment had a different effect. Before beginning each application the circuits had to be tuned, using the electrodes to be used for that treatment. Changing the size of the electrode altered the tuning. When using the labile electrodes and altering the area of electrode in contact with the patient the frequency as well as the intensity of current was altered. With the modern automatic tuning this no longer happens as the frequency is kept constant. In this case it is a pity, as better results were obtained when the frequency altered as the pads were moved, but on the other hand the tuning for each application was difficult and time-consuming.

Three-times-toleration

This is a method of treating a localised condition in which the tender area is actually anaesthetised. A 100Hz current is selected. Two very small electrodes or the very tips of the labile electrodes are used. The site of tenderness is located and the electrodes placed where the patient feels the current most intensely. The success of the treatment depends on accurate siting. The intensity is increased until the patient feels a most intense prickling, as strong as he can tolerate; this is usually accompanied by a muscular contraction. The pads are kept absolutely still until the muscle relaxes and the prickling begins to die away. The current is then increased again to tolerance. This is repeated a third time, then the current is turned down and off before the pads are removed. If the pads are removed without decreasing the current it is extremely uncomfortable for the patient, it feels as if the skin is being torn off. Also it is difficult to remove the pad cleanly and not slip to a new area of skin.

If the pad is moved after the *first* increase of current, the new area of skin is receiving more than the highest tolerance of the patient, and is very painful indeed. For this reason it is essential when using this method that the operator, as well as the patient, is comfortable, and able to reach both the apparatus and the area to be treated without stretching. If the pads gradually slide into a new position the prickling does not die away, the tetanic contraction of the muscle does not relax and anaesthesia will not be produced. The patient will be enduring considerable discomfort for nothing.

The success of this treatment depends on the co-operation of the patient. The hypersensitive patient will not tolerate enough current to achieve any effect; the patient who endures past reasonable discomfort under the mistaken impression that 'the more he endures the better the effect will be' will suffer from after-pain. The patient who will tell the operator when the point of discomfort but not agony is reached will get excellent relief of pain. The operator must watch for the tetanic contraction of the muscle. As soon as this is produced the current is kept steady until a rhythmical relaxation and contraction begins and the patient reports being comfortable; only then may the current be increased for the second, then the third time. After the third increase the muscle should be allowed to relax completely before ceasing treatment.

'TRIGGER POINTS'

The tender areas are not always the site of the lesions but are sometimes 'trigger points' at some distance from the affected part but having the same autonomic nerve supply. The trigger point is not necessarily in the same spinal segment as the affected organ, as autonomic connections run both up and down the ganglionic chain. Nevertheless, treatment of such trigger points will often produce an effect on the distant structure (probably by influencing the circulation) leading to an immediate relief of pain usually but not always temporary, and accelerated resolution of the lesion.

REMOTE CONTROL

To facilitate turning up the current while holding the pads stationary a remote control may be used. This may be a foot control operated by the physiotherapist, or a hand control by the patient. The intensity control of the apparatus is set to a maximum which cannot then be exceeded by operation of the remote control. This is a safety precaution to prevent the patient overdosing himself. The control is given to the patient and the operator then has both hands free to manipulate the electrodes. Care must be taken to see that he understands that he is to make only three clean increases of current, stopping each time at the point of toleration. He must not continually turn up the current a little. If he does so, a satisfactory anaesthesia is not produced. If the patient cannot be relied on to obey instructions the control must be operated by another member of staff.

When the pads are removed the part treated is found to be almost if not totally anaesthetic. There may, rarely, be a transient period of hyperaesthesia followed by anaesthesia. When sensation returns after a period of seconds or minutes the part will appear to have normal sensation and be no longer tender. Often one treatment will be enough to banish the tenderness permanently, but if it returns the treatment may be repeated next day or as required.

It is important to stress moderation in this treatment. It is uncomfortable, but not excessively so, and attempts on the part of the patient to be 'tough' are counterproductive.

After giving an anaesthetising dose to an injured ligament or torn muscle it is important not to leave it unsupported, or, with no protective pain, the injury may be reproduced. Efficient strapping is essential. Further, if manipulation is to be performed it should be done after the general relaxing treatment but before the three-times-toleration treatment, or it is the equivalent of manipulation under anaesthetic. The strong dose following manipulation relieves the residual soreness.

4. Treatment with Interferential Therapy

It cannot be emphasised too strongly that there is no such thing as a routine application of interferential therapy. At each treatment the following questions must be considered:

1. What do I hope to achieve?
2. How can this best be done?
3. What frequency would be most effective?
4. Is a sweep of frequencies required?
5. Should treatment be general, local or both?
6. Should two or four electrodes be used?
7. Where exactly are the electrodes to be placed?
8. How long a treatment should be given?

Having made a decision about these at the first treatment it does not necessarily follow that the next application would be identical. Other questions arise:

1. What was the effect of the last treatment?
2. In what way has the condition changed, and what changes if any must therefore be made in the application?
3. Was the relief of pain not satisfactory? The treatment may have been (a) too short; (b) too long; or (c) too strong a local dose.
4. Was the wrong area treated, either from error of diagnosis or, worse, careless application of electrodes, with more attention to ease of application than to accuracy?
5. Was the patient excessively tired after treatment, due to too long a session, or, possibly, due to the operator yielding to the patient's request that the treatment be continued as 'the pain is going'?

6. Was the relief of pain short lived? The placing of the electrodes was then correct, but a longer or stronger treatment would have been more effective. When there is any relief, however short, it can confidently be predicted that after the next treatment it will be more prolonged.

INTENSITY OF TREATMENT

Except for the three-times-toleration dose interferential therapy is comfortable. The intensity of current used is one which produces a strong but comfortable prickling but no muscular contraction. The current is increased until the patient feels a definite prickling. It is left at this intensity until the prickling dies away – about one minute. It is then increased until the patient reports a slight muscular contraction, and then decreased until the contraction subsides. This is then the correct intensity of current. Unless the point of contraction is reached there is no means of assessing what intensity is 'just short' of that necessary to produce a contraction and the patient would therefore receive too mild a treatment to produce any effects.

When using vacuum electrodes the patient may be confused as to whether he can feel a contraction or not. To help him appreciate the feeling allow him to become accustomed to the tightening and release of the suction cups; apply a minimal current until he is used to the prickling; turn up the current until he feels a tightening of the muscle quite distinct from the suction; decrease the current until he feels no tightening in the muscle. This is the correct intensity for the treatment despite the fact that he will become accustomed to the prickling and, after about 10 minutes, probably feel nothing at all.

In very acute cases the patient may feel discomfort at a very low intensity of current. In this case no attempt is made to increase the intensity but a longer treatment is given. Very rarely in such a case would a three-times-toleration dose be attempted.

DURATION OF TREATMENT

As a rule treatment is short, beginning with 10–15 minutes except in the acute case as mentioned above. Treatment at a normal intensity should not be given to one area for longer than 20 minutes. If more than one area is to be treated the total time should not exceed 30 minutes. Too long a treatment makes the patient unacceptably tired later in the day.

FREQUENCY OF TREATMENT

In most cases it is desirable that treatment be given daily for five days. Initially, relief of pain is short but becomes longer after each successive treatment. After five days the relief probably lasts from one treatment to the next. As soon as this happens the treatment is given every other day and then, as soon as the relief is continuous again, every third day. A course of 12 treatments suffices in most cases.

If this plan is not feasible, treatment is given every other day from the beginning but it will take longer to achieve a cure. Treatment less than twice a week is usually a waste of time.

There are, of course, exceptions to this general plan. For instance, in the treatment of incontinence, because the muscle requires time to re-establish its tone, no useful purpose is served by treating daily. Three times a week is the ideal but twice a week is adequate.

LENGTH OF COURSE

In general, a course of 12 treatments is sufficient. When dealing with long-standing conditions this may not be enough, and there is no reason why treatment should not be continued, providing progress is being made. It is not to be expected that if a condition, such as post-herpetic neuralgia, has persisted for 10 years it will disappear within a month. If the patient becomes over-tired with prolonged treatment, it should be suspended and resumed after a month.

CONTRA-INDICATIONS

There are comparatively few absolute contra-indications to interferential therapy.

THROMBOSIS

It is said that the current produces chemical changes in the blood leading to alterations in the clotting time; at present there is no hard evidence to support this. Treatment must not be given to any patient who is taking anticoagulants as it renders these ineffective. The effect of the current is on the platelets and would tend to spread any clot with perhaps fatal results in a patient with coronary thrombosis. If a patient has a history of deep vein thrombosis, even many years past, the treatment may increase rather than decrease swelling.

PACEMAKERS

Patients with pacemakers should avoid all high and medium frequency generators.

CARDIAC CONDITIONS

The electrodes should be placed to avoid the stellate ganglion and the heart itself.

BACTERIAL INFECTIONS

The effect on bacteria is uncertain, and it is advisable that bacterial infections should not be treated, unless there is open drainage.

MALIGNANCY

It has not been proved that interferential therapy has any

accelerating effect on malignancy. It certainly may be used to relieve referred pain.

SHORT WAVE DIATHERMY

The interferential therapy apparatus must be at least 6 metres (20ft) from a short wave diathermy machine (preferably in another room) or the circuit may be damaged and the patient could experience a sudden surge of current when the short wave diathermy machine is turned off (see p. 34).

5. Treatment of Recent Injuries

Interferential therapy is often the treatment of choice for recent injuries. It should be initiated at the earliest possible moment to produce the most rapid and satisfactory result; clinically, there appears to be no danger of increasing bleeding or bruising.

As there is no concentration of current on areas deficient in the stratum corneum, treatment may be given without pain even if the skin is broken, though if the electrode is placed on an abraded area, sterile precautions must be observed.

Because a badly bruised area may be painful due to the pressure caused by bandaging on an electrode, the four-electrode method should be used; the electrodes being placed above and below the affected part and directing the current through it. If there is no undue tenderness then the two-electrode method may be used.

AIMS OF TREATMENT

1. To relieve pain.
2. To reduce swelling.
3. To promote healing.
4. To restore function.

Relief of pain

Relief of pain is of first importance not only as an end in itself but because pain produces spasm, unnatural movement and production of further strains. However, it must not be forgotten that spasm may be protective and its removal may leave the injured structure open to repetition of the original injury. Therefore when spasm has been relieved, support must be given with bandage or strapping to prevent uncontrolled or excessive range of movement. This must also follow if an anaesthetising dose is part of the treatment.

METHOD

Using the four-electrode method the site of injury is located; two electrodes are placed immediately above and two below so that the currents cross at the site of injury. The electrodes should be as large as can comfortably be accommodated as this allows a greater intensity of current to be passed without discomfort. In a tapered limb it may be necessary to use smaller electrodes below the injury than above, but as each circuit has one large and one small electrode they are still in balance.

A constant frequency in the sedative range (100–130Hz) is selected; 130Hz being the most effective if this is available. The current intensity is increased to produce a definite prickling well within the patient's tolerance and allowed to flow for 15–20 minutes or even longer if the spasm is not relieved.

If a single point of acute tenderness can be located, a strong dose may be given to anaesthetise the part but this may well not be indicated at the first treatment. This is best administered as a three-times-toleration dose using the labile electrodes but if the apparatus does not allow this the stud electrode is used to pass the maximum current the patient can tolerate for three minutes.

Either treatment produces a numbing effect so strapping is applied immediately and correct movement taught. Prolonged exercise must be avoided for at least an hour. The longer the period of rest between treatment and exercise, the longer the freedom from pain will last. In hospital this rest period is often difficult to achieve because of pressure on space in the department. At subsequent attendances the re-education and exercises should be given *before* the interferential therapy, and the patient encouraged to have a considerable rest period before doing his home exercises.

At the second treatment, checking the movements gives a good assessment of the effect of the first treatment. The strapping need not be removed unless reduction of swelling has made it slack and ineffective. Electrodes can be placed above and below the strapping, as removal of the strapping at each attendance will only cause discomfort and unnecessary wear and tear on the skin.

If the part is still very painful and spasm has returned treatment is given exactly as the first treatment (previously described).

If the patient reports that there was not even transitory relief the position of the electrodes should be varied as, clearly, the crossing of the currents had not been at the correct place.

If the pain is less and the spasm reduced, treatment is given in the analgesic range (100–130Hz) constant for 10 minutes followed by a small sweep, say of 10Hz, round 100–130Hz.

Treatment is then repeated daily, gradually increasing both extent and duration of the sweep as the condition improves until the patient is receiving 10 minutes' constant analgesic and a 10 minutes' sweep of 10–100Hz. If it is found that introducing the sweep increases the pain, or the relief of pain is not as satisfactory, treatment is given with analgesic frequency only for two or three days before trying once more to introduce the sweep. Daily treatment is given until the pain does not return significantly between treatments, then dropped to alternate days.

An area which is not unduly sensitive to pressure may be treated in exactly the same way using the two-electrode method. In this case, one electrode is placed immediately over the lesion and a larger directing electrode ideally placed opposite it or, in some sites, a co-planar treatment may be preferable. This treatment is often less comfortable, but is easier to place accurately. The directing electrode is moved over the part until the pain is exacerbated and then secured in this position, as the increase of pain indicates that the current is passing through the site of injury. The pattern of treatment is exactly as that for the four-electrode method. Obviously the two-electrode technique cannot be employed once strapping has been applied to the part, but can be reverted to on the days the strapping has to be removed.

Reduction of bruising and swelling

Reduction and/or removal of bruising and swelling, with minimum delay, is important because organisation of the exudate leads to the formation of adhesions and impairment of function.

Since no passive congestion is produced by interferential therapy it is possible to institute treatment immediately after injury without risk of haemorrhage. If the skin is broken there is no increase of exudate, but care must be taken to avoid introducing any infection.

A constant analgesic current is used initially while the bruise is painful followed by a sweep increasing to 10–100Hz as soon as possible as this is the major part of the treatment. Frequencies of 10–150Hz stimulating the parasympathetic nerves increase the blood flow through the part assisting in resolution. The contractions of voluntary muscle which are produced by the lower frequencies assist in the dispersal of excess fluid. For this reason the intensity of current is slightly greater when using the sweep than for the constant frequency. While it would be contra-indicated to allow a muscular contraction at 100Hz constant (because such a held contraction would cause after-pain), when using a sweep the intensity should be such that a contraction is just produced in the lower frequencies to which the voluntary muscles are most sensitive, but relaxation in the higher frequencies where a stronger current would be required.

The colour of the bruise will be seen to change from the first treatment, though deep and extensive bruising, or a haematoma, may take several weeks to disperse. This method of treatment may safely be employed where there is bruising of the thigh or the brachialis muscles when other treatments are contra-indicated for fear of inducing myositis ossificans. Indeed it has been reported that a case of myositis ossificans which had been confirmed radiographically, and treatment by interferential therapy was continued, cleared completely with no calcification being demonstrable after three weeks.

If it is possible to do so on the apparatus available, the lowest frequencies, 0–5Hz, should be cut out to avoid stimulation of the sympathetic nerves.

Promotion of healing

While the method by which healing is accelerated is obscure it can be observed clinically that recovery is assisted. This may be because of the active increase of circulation, but probably also by altering the electrical state of the cell which has been changed by injury.

Restoration of function

When there is noticeable muscle wasting, treatment may be given in addition with a sweep of 5–50Hz with a view to stimulating the striped muscle. If the apparatus will not produce this range the nearest selection to it has to suffice. It will be noted that while a sweep of 0–100Hz is applied, for a proportion of the time the patient will be receiving the lower frequencies which stimulate the muscle. The object of giving the extra dose in the lower frequencies only is to enhance the effect. To increase the effect the electrodes should be moved for this part of the treatment so that the *belly of the affected muscle* lies in the path of the interference current, *not the site of the injury*. In many cases it is more convenient to stimulate the muscle with the faradic rather than the interferential current.

(Recent work in Holland suggests that the strengthening of striped muscle is more pronounced if the carrying frequency of the interference current is 2000Hz instead of 4000Hz. Some apparatus now includes the facility for applying this current.)

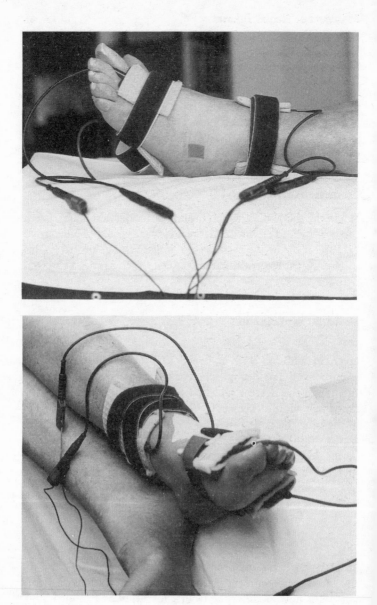

Treatment with interferential therapy does not replace, but only augments, re-education of muscles and exercises.

By applying these principles the treatment for an individual injury may be decided. In the following illustrations, a likely method of application is shown. There is no one 'correct' method; each case must be assessed (Figs. 5/1, 5/2, 5/3, 5/4, 5/5, 5/6, 5/7, 5/8. See also Fig. 3/13).

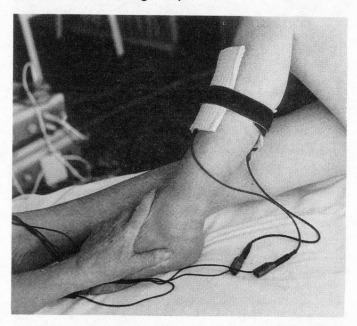

Fig. 5/3 Ruptured fibres of calf muscle treated using the bi-polar method

---

Fig. 5/1 (*top left*) Sprained left ankle: electrode arrangement to treat the point indicated

Fig. 5/2 (*bottom left*) Treatment to a sprained left ankle which is strapped

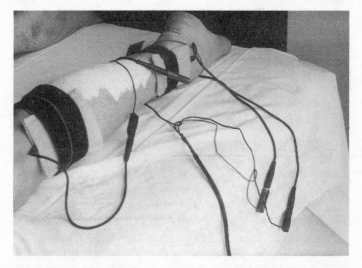

Fig. 5/4   Ruptured fibres of calf muscle being treated with strapping in place

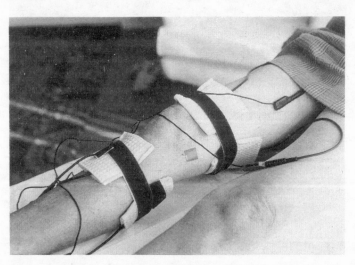

Fig. 5/5   Treatment of strained medial ligament of right knee

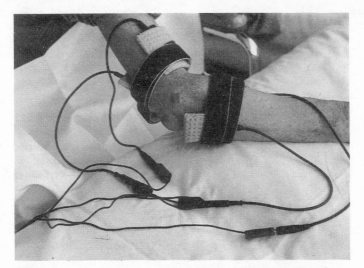

Fig. 5/6   Tennis elbow: one method of electrode arrangement

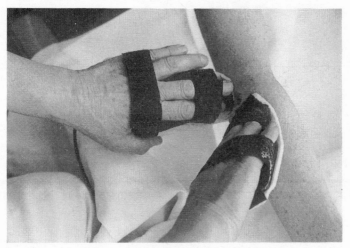

Fig. 5/7   Localised treatment of tennis elbow using labile electrodes

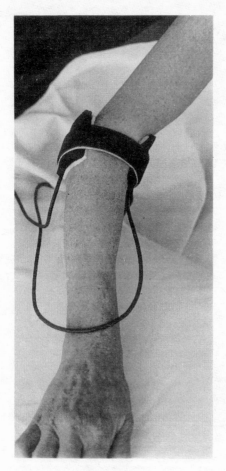

Fig. 5/8 Tennis elbow: alternative method of electrode arrangement

6. Treatment of Herpes Zoster

Although modern drugs have revolutionised the treatment of the acute phase of herpes zoster (shingles), post-herpetic neuralgia remains a common sequel. There are many patients who have suffered an intractable neuralgia for many years, and even these people are not beyond hope of recovery. Although it is desirable to begin treatment as soon as the scabs are shed, as this produces the most rapid response, it is well worthwhile to treat a patient with a history extending over years. In this case a rapid result cannot be expected, but the pain becomes less acute after one or two treatments, and pain-free periods lengthen progressively as the treatment continues. As well as relieving the pain, the current has the effect of reducing the scarring.

The whole area originally affected is usually covered with unsightly white puckered scars. These are obvious as soon as the scabs are shed and do not improve markedly as the years go by. As treatment proceeds the scars begin to flatten out and become pigmented so that they are much less obvious. The patient is delighted with the relief of pain, but this is a bonus, particularly with facial scarring. It has been found that corneal scarring is affected in the same way. Patients with herpes affecting the ophthalmic branch of the trigeminal nerve often have interference with vision due to the scarring distorting the cornea. After a few treatments the patient reports that the vision is clearing. Normal vision may not be achieved, but any improvement is acceptable.

For the patient with a recent attack of herpes zoster, treatment is begun as soon as possible after the scabs have been shed. Treatment before this is not advisable because of the risk of infection spread. Treatment is begun cautiously as the response to the current is likely to be exaggerated owing to the recent inflammation of the nerve. Using the four-electrode method the pads are placed so that the whole course of the affected nerve lies in the path of the current. This is simple enough in the case of a limb, but requires special techniques for the trigeminal nerve or thoracic nerve.

The thoracic nerve cannot be treated in one application. If the pads are placed on the origin and distal end of a thoracic nerve the current would simply take the shortest pathway through the chest and not pass along the nerve (Fig. 6/1a). Two applications must be made: one using the pads placed X and Y, and the

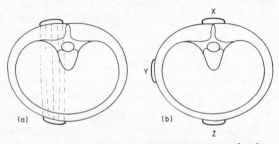

Fig. 6/1   Application of interferential current for the
treatment of a thoracic nerve: (a) wrong; (b) right

second application using the pads placed Y and Z (Fig. 6/1b). The current is thus directed along the posterior and anterior parts of the nerve. Figure 6/2 shows the application of the electrodes for this treatment.

A constant frequency in the sedative range (100–130Hz) is chosen. A very low intensity, just perceptible, is passed for 5–10 minutes. The patient may report at first that the pain is intensified, but this is not a contra-indication as this sensation will reduce while the current is flowing, and be absent when the current is turned off. The pads are then placed so that the currents cross through the nerve cells of the dorsal root ganglion of the affected segment, and a further 5–10 minutes' sedative

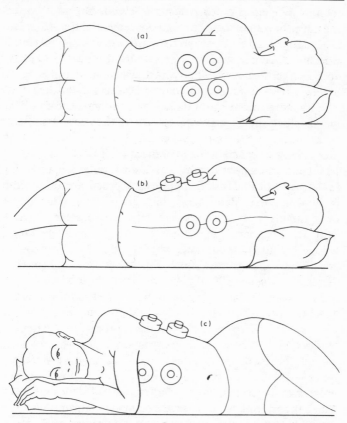

Fig. 6/2 Position of the electrodes for treating a thoracic nerve: (a) treating the nerve root; (b) treating the posterior half of the nerve distribution; (c) treating the anterior half of the nerve distribution

treatment given. At the next treatment, provided that the patient reports some improvement even if only marginal or transient, the time and, later, the intensity are increased according to progress. Treatment is given daily for five days at least, then dropped to alternate days as the pain relief lasts longer and then to twice weekly. Treatment may be stopped as soon as the pain is much reduced or cured, but may have to continue for some time if the commencement of treatment has been delayed. After three weeks, particularly if the patient is elderly or in poor health, he may report being unduly tired in the evening after treatment. This is not unusual, but it may be wiser to have a week or fortnight free of treatment and then resume.

With more chronic cases there may be adherent scars which increase the pain. Treatment is given with the electrodes placed as before, using an intensity of current only just short of producing a contraction for 7–10 minutes. This is followed by 10 minutes' sweep, beginning with a small range (about 10Hz) in the region of 100Hz so that the greater proportion of the time is still within the sedative range, only gradually introducing the more stimulating frequencies so that the nerve is not irritated. If pain after treatment is increased, the sweep is maintained for a few treatments at the last range which produced no irritation. If you are using apparatus which will not produce a gradually increasing range, the 90–100Hz sweep must be used for four or five treatments before going on to the 0–100Hz sweep. It is the lower frequencies which produce the slight muscle contraction which assists in stretching the scar tissue producing a flattening of the scars, but these frequencies cannot be employed too soon without the risk of irritating the nerve. Treatment is given three times a week for four weeks or longer if necessary. As treatment progresses the scars gradually flatten and fade. In some cases where the scarring has been severe enough to impair function it is possible by this treatment to restore movement even after a lapse of years.

When the trigeminal nerve is affected it is almost impossible to apply four separate electrodes. The small combined four-stud electrode may be used but this covers so small an area that several applications must be made to cover the affected part. The pair of stud electrodes used together gives a somewhat better coverage. Both these applications have the disadvantage of allowing the passage of very little current.

If the apparatus allows, a better method is to use the two-

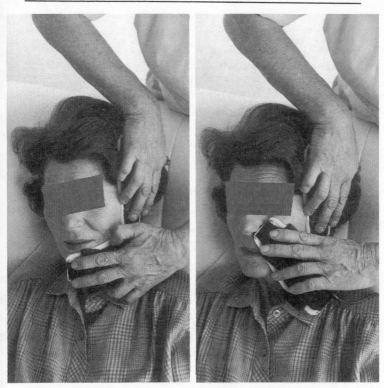

Fig. 6/3 (*left*) Post-herpetic neuralgia of the trigeminal nerve. Position of electrodes using the labile method for treating the mandibular branch
Fig. 6/4 (*right*) As Fig. 6/3, but treating the maxillary branch

electrode method with labile electrodes (Figs. 6/3, 6/4, 6/5). One is placed over the point of emergence of the nerve and the other moved slowly over the course of the nerve using only the tip of the electrode. The current is increased until the patient reports a definite tingling and as the pad moves indicates any point where the current feels stronger. When the tender area is reached the pad is kept still until the prickling dies away and then moved on. When the pad passes over the area again it will be found to be no

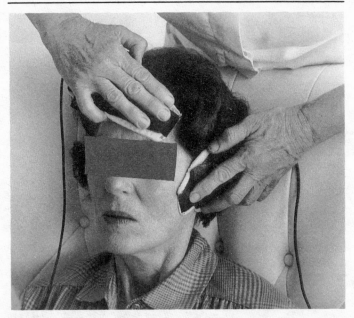

Fig. 6/5   As Fig. 6/3, but treating the ophthalmic branch

more sensitive than the surrounding tissue. When the whole area has been treated the current is turned down and the pad removed.

Particular care is needed when treating the *ophthalmic* branch (Fig. 6/5). The current will feel much stronger where there is so little tissue overlying the bone; therefore, on passing from the lower to the upper part of the face, the current should be reduced. When there is much pain in the eye itself the pads are not placed on the eyelid but the eye is treated from *two* directions: firstly with one pad on the forehead immediately above the eye and the other below the eye; and, secondly, with one pad on the bridge of the nose and the other on the temple. In this way the whole of the cornea receives treatment. It cannot be denied that this treatment is far from comfortable but the relief obtained from the moment the current is turned off makes it acceptable to the patient. The duration of this relief becomes progressively longer. For treatment of *pain* a constant sedative frequency is used; if *scarring of the cornea* is also being treated a short period (2–5 minutes) of a small range sweep may be added. Treatment lasts 10–15 minutes and is repeated three times a week.

Exactly the same method may be used for the treatment of *trigeminal neuralgia* not associated with herpes zoster. Success has been obtained in cases which were so severe that removal of the trigeminal ganglion had been contemplated. In such cases a three-times-toleration dose was also given to the most tender spot.

7. Treatment of Rheumatic Conditions

Interferential therapy is the treatment of choice for all types of rheumatic conditions. It can be used effectively in the acute and chronic stages of rheumatoid arthritis, in osteoarthritis and spondylitis.

RHEUMATOID ARTHRITIS

The aims of treatment are threefold: the relief of pain; decrease of inflammation; and increase of range of movement. Restoration of function is taken care of by other means. The relative priorities vary with the phase of the disease.

Acute phase

In the acute phase the prime consideration is the relief of pain and swelling. Treatment is given usually by the four-electrode method to avoid causing pressure on the painful joint. The electrodes are placed well above and below the joint to include a wide area. If an acutely inflamed joint is resting in plaster of Paris splints, treatment may still be given with the electrodes in this position. Usually plate electrodes are more comfortable than vacuum cups but unless the contours of the patient make application of the cups impossible, the choice should rest with the patient; it makes no difference to the efficiency of treatment. The largest electrodes that can be accommodated are used to give the deepest possible penetration. A constant sedative (100 or 130Hz) current is passed for 10 minutes at a comfortable tingling intensity but short of producing any contraction. Too great an intensity causing contraction will certainly cause after-pain and must be avoided.

If there is any doubt about the patient's appreciation of what is required it is better to underdose rather than overdose at this stage. Care must be taken to ensure that the patient understands the difference between the 'tightening' of the vacuum which is inevitable and the 'tightening' of the muscle which must be avoided (see p. 53). Provided this is understood the treatment will give relief even in the most acute phase of the disease, when the joints are red, shiny and swollen. The relief may be short lived at first, but treatment is repeated daily and freedom from pain increases at each treatment. In most cases it will shorten the acute phase. Duration of treatment is increased to 20 minutes but the current is kept low until the acute phase has passed.

Chronic phase

In the chronic phase, in addition to the sedative treatment, it is desirable to treat with those frequencies which influence the blood vessels and muscles. The 10 minutes' analgesic treatment is followed by a period of sweep. In the subacute phase the sweep is introduced gradually, beginning with a sweep of 20–30Hz just below the sedative frequency (e.g. if a 130Hz current was used for the acute phase, the sweep would be 100–120/130Hz) for three or four minutes according to the condition of the patient and increasing both range and duration until a sweep of 10–100Hz is being given for 10 minutes. This progression depends on the report of the patient as to improvement and the observable improvement in the condition of the joint. If the patient presents in the chronic phase, the full sweep may be introduced at once. The intensity of current is such that it just fails to produce a contraction for the constant treatment, but during the sweep produces a contraction only as the optimum frequency for stimulation of the motor nerves is reached, followed by relaxation for the rest of the cycle.

In addition to the local application, treatment is also given to

that region of the spine from which the joint is innervated.
Using the four-electrode method, five to seven minutes'
treatment is given with a sweep of 10–100Hz sweep. This is to
stimulate the autonomic nerves affecting the blood supply to the
joint, producing an active increase in circulation. The effect is
quite different from that of the electrical treatments, such as
short wave diathermy, which are often given. These treatments,
by producing heat and so a passive congestion in and around the
joint, cause increased exudate and consequently increased
tension in an already tense joint; this causes an increase of pain
and improvement is felt only after a time. The active congestion
produced by the interferential therapy causes an increased rate
of blood flow, absorption of increased exudate and decreased
tension. The patient therefore leaves the department already
feeling more comfortable. The additional time spent at each
attendance in treating the spine is well compensated for by the
decreased number of attendances required to produce the
desired results.

OSTEOARTHRITIS OF THE HIP JOINT
(Figs. 7/1, 7/2)

Treatment of the osteoarthritic hip is particularly rewarding.
The patient is treated in crook side lying on the good side with
the affected leg supported on a pillow. This is a comfortable
position for most patients. Vacuum electrodes of medium size
are used if available; plate electrodes are possible but are more
difficult to secure in position. The lower electrodes are placed
opposite each other on the front and back of the thigh just below
the ischial tuberosity. The upper ones are placed one anteriorly
on the abdomen just above the centre of the inguinal ligament
and the other on the back opposite (Fig. 7/1). The two currents
then cross in the hip joint. Seven minutes' constant sedative
frequency (100 or 130Hz) is given followed by seven minutes'
10–100Hz sweep. With the patient in the same position the

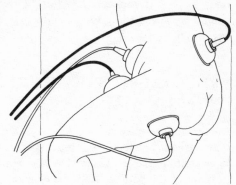

Fig. 7/1   OA hip
treated using vacuum
electrodes

Fig. 7/2   OA hip: treating
the lumbar spine as an
adjunct to the hip treatment

electrodes are moved to treat the lumbo-sacral spine with a
sweep of 10–100Hz for seven minutes (Fig. 7/2). After
treatment the patient should rest for at least 10 minutes,
preferably longer, and undertake no severe exercises for at least
an hour. The longer the rest period, the longer the relief of pain
will last. If an exercise class is to be undertaken this must
precede, not follow, treatment. Immediately after treatment the
patient has less pain and the range of movement is increased.
This may last only a short time at first but is more prolonged
after each treatment. Treatment is given two or three times a
week for 12 treatments. Daily treatment is not necessary, but

once a week is ineffective. After 12 treatments the patient should cease attending for a month to prevent him becoming over-tired.

OSTEOARTHRITIS OF THE KNEE JOINT
(Figs. 7/3, 7/4)

In treating the knee it cannot be over-emphasised how much better are the results if the lumbar spine is treated as well as the knee joint. This is not as convenient as with the hip because the position of the patient has to be changed; for this reason it is often, regrettably, omitted. As with the hip the maximum effect on the circulation is achieved through the autonomic supply arising in the lumbar spine.

With the knee joint it is also possible to vary the position of the electrodes from one treatment to another so as to be certain

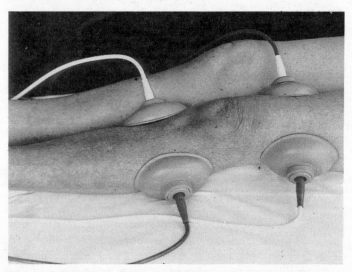

Fig. 7/3   OA knee treated with the electrodes placed laterally above and below the joint

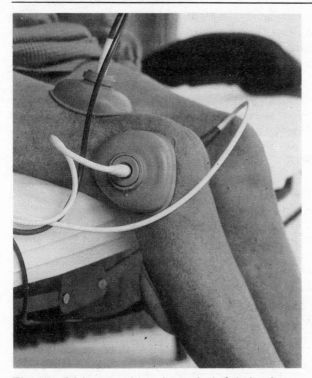

Fig. 7/4 OA knee: an alternative method of placing the electrodes. Also used for treating the cruciate ligaments

that all aspects of the joint are treated. Thus one treatment may be given with the electrodes placed laterally, one pair above the knee, and one pair below the knee (Fig. 7/3). At the next treatment they are placed anteriorly and posteriorly above and below the knee; while at the next session the patient can be sitting with the knee flexed, one circuit traversing the knee from side to side and the other from the suprapatellar pouch to the calf, as in the treatment of the cruciate ligaments (Fig. 7/4).

While the most effective position can be found for each patient, variations should always be tried to achieve the best result. Some patients find that treatment with the two-electrode method is more effective. Here, one pad is placed over the most painful area and the other directly opposite directing the already modulated current straight through the joint. The patient usually reports that the current is 'picking out the painful spot'; if he does not the electrode is moved until he does. The increased pain dies away after a few minutes and relief persists after treatment. Why some patients respond to the two-electrode method rather than the four is obscure and unpredictable, but in any one patient it is remarkably constant over the years.

Some patients, even in the chronic stage, find relief from the constant current but increased pain if any sweep is introduced. In this case the whole treatment, 15 minutes, is given with the sedative current and a good result is obtained but more slowly. Treatment to the spine with a sweep may be tolerated; if not, the constant frequency is applied here also.

Arthritic patients are often elderly, and may have a cardiac condition which is not associated with the arthritis. In such cases treatment to the spine, even in the sitting position, may cause respiratory distress due to too great an alteration of the circulation. These patients must be watched carefully; at the first sign of distress, however slight, treatment to the spine must be stopped. In some cases it may be advisable not to treat the spine even though the relief of pain will be less effective and recovery slower.

ANKYLOSING SPONDYLITIS

Interferential therapy is also effective in relieving the persistent aching of ankylosing spondylitis. When the pain is diffuse the four-electrode method is used, treating a wide field with large electrodes to get maximum penetration. Treatment is given for 10 minutes with a constant sedative current (100 or 130Hz) at an intensity just short of producing a contraction, followed by 10 minutes' sweep of 10–100Hz. Treatment is given three times a week for a month, followed by a rest of two or three weeks. Interferential therapy must be combined with exercises which encourage extension, performed either before or some hours after the treatment. Pain is reduced and range of movement improved. Most spondylitic patients require a course of treatment two or three times a year to maintain movement.

SPONDYLOSIS (SPINAL OSTEOARTHRITIS)

Spondylosis or osteoarthritis of the spine is particularly suitable for interferential therapy. Patients often respond to this when all else has failed. If the pain is diffuse the whole area is treated as for spondylitis (above). After a few treatments the patient usually reports some localisation of the pain. This may be verified by using either the glove or the four-stud electrode. These are placed on the skin at a point of normal sensation and the current increased to produce a slight prickling. The electrodes are then moved, gradually working towards the pain enquiring if the sensation is less, the same, or more at each point. As the electrode is applied to the tender point the current feels stronger, though the intensity is the same. When the most tender point is identified, treatment is given with constant frequency and sweep centred at this point. After treatment the localised current is again applied. It may be found that the point is no longer tender, but if tenderness persists the point is treated with a strong local dose with the stud electrode or a three-times-toleration dose, according to the apparatus available. A course of up to 12 treatments is usually given two or three times a week. The local dose is only given when indicated, not as a routine.

CERVICAL SPONDYLOSIS (Fig. 7/5)

Treatment of cervical spondylosis is satisfactory if care is taken, but there are difficulties. The most common error is to omit the upper joints by placing the electrodes on the neck itself. The atlanto-occipital and atlanto-axial joints lie above the hair line, so it is impossible to attach vacuum electrodes. Plate electrodes are placed on either side of the occiput and the two lower electrodes just below the vertebra prominens (spine of the seventh cervical vertebra). Bandaging is difficult, but if the patient is treated in half lying the upper electrodes may be kept in place with a towel round the neck and a soft pillow as a 'butterfly' tucked in each side of the neck.

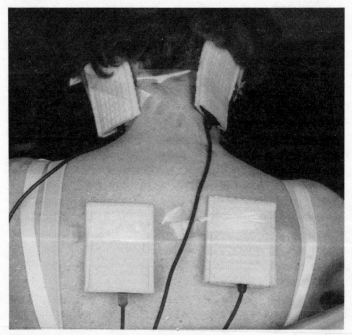

Fig. 7/5   Treatment of cervical spondylosis

MUSCULAR PAIN

Patients with widespread muscular pains over the shoulder girdle will often respond best to labile treatment only. Using the glove electrodes and a 100Hz current of an intensity to produce definite prickling, the electrodes are moved over the whole shoulder girdle. Both electrodes may be moved at once, or one kept stationary and the other moved whichever may be done most smoothly by the operator. As the pad passes over a tender area the current is felt more intensely, and the pad is kept on this spot until it is no longer tender. The operator then moves on to the next tender spot until the whole area has been treated. On returning to the first tender spots they will now be found to be quite normal. The relief of pain may last hours, days or weeks, and treatment is repeated as necessary.

SEPTIC ARTHRITIS

Following septic arthritis the patient is often left with gross and intractable stiffness. Treatment with any form of heat is contra-indicated in case of residual infection but with interferential therapy practically no heat is produced.

The joint is treated from as many aspects as possible. Treatment is given daily beginning with 10 minutes' constant sedative current at a very low intensity to relieve pain. This is increased slowly to 20 minutes. If there is no increase of pain, or any sign of a flare-up, the duration of the constant frequency is progressively decreased and replaced by gradually increasing sweep until the patient is receiving 10 minutes' sedative treatment and 10 minutes' sweep of 10–100Hz. As this treatment stretches and releases scarring of the skin so the fibrous tissue within the joint becomes pliable and the range of movement is gradually restored. Daily treatment may be given but a rapid result cannot be expected. Perseverance,

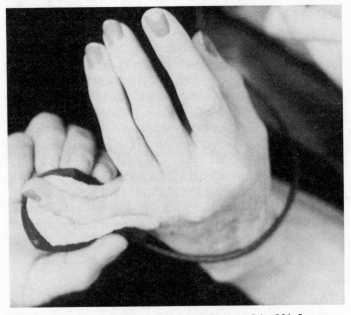

Fig. 7/6 OA affecting the interphalangeal joints of the fifth finger
being treated by a small stud electrode wrapped round the finger

accompanied by an increasing programme of exercise, can
restore full range of movement.

ARTHRITIS AFFECTING THE HANDS

Single interphalangeal joints of finger or thumb, the metacarpo-
phalangeal joint of the thumb, and Heberden's nodes which
have become painful and swollen are most conveniently treated
using the small stud electrode wrapped round the finger (Fig.
7/6). The current which can be passed is small but is adequate
for the superficial joints. The frequencies and timings are as for
any other rheumatic joint.

In the case of the inflamed Heberden's nodes, sedative treatment (100 or 130Hz) only is used. Relief of pain is almost immediate and the hand can be used normally. Two or three treatments may suffice to restore painless function. The nodes will still be present but will no longer incommode the patient. Treatment is repeated as necessary.

8. Treatment of Shoulder Pain

A frozen shoulder is one of the most troublesome conditions to treat because of the diversity of causes. The importance of accurate diagnosis and localisation of the site of the lesion cannot be stressed too strongly; if it is not, then much time will be wasted. The trouble may lie in the subdeltoid bursa (Fig. 8/1), the rotator cuff or the biceps brachii tendon (Fig. 8/2), or a generalised capsulitis may be present (Fig. 8/3). Supraspinatus tendinitis may present a similar picture (Fig. 8/4).

It is clear that when using a treatment which depends for its effect on the crossing of the two currents at the site of the lesion localisation is of paramount importance.

The four-electrode method is generally used. As a general rule, plate electrodes are preferable to the vacuum cups, as most shoulders have too many bony prominences to allow cups to be sited accurately. On a large well-covered shoulder, small vacuum electrodes may be possible, but on the thin patient, or one with bulging muscles, pads held by a crêpe bandage allow a more accurate application. Small pads about 5cm (2in) square are used. It is not satisfactory to use the small combined electrode as far too little current can be tolerated; the distribution of current is too small and too superficial to have much effect.

A constant sedative current (100 or 130Hz) is passed for 10 minutes. If the condition is acute, the time may be increased at subsequent treatments up to 20 minutes until the condition becomes subacute. The pads are then moved to treat the cervical spine for 10 minutes with a sweep of 10–100Hz. If available the labile electrodes are used to treat the deltoid, trapezius and infraspinatus muscles with a frequency of 10–50Hz at an

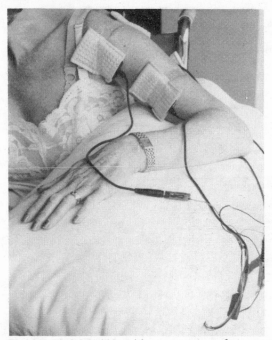

Fig. 8/1 Subdeltoid bursitis: arrangement of electrodes

intensity to produce a slight contraction. At subsequent treatments the period of constant frequency is reduced and replaced by a sweep gradually increasing to 10–100Hz. When the generalised pain is decreased but local pain remains, this point is given either a strong dose with the stud electrode for three minutes or a three-times-toleration dose with the glove electrodes.

Treatment is given daily for five days or until the pain does not reappear between treatments, then dropped to three times a week for one week, then twice a week. In recent cases 12 treatments may suffice, but long-standing cases take considerably longer. After four weeks a change of treatment should be considered.

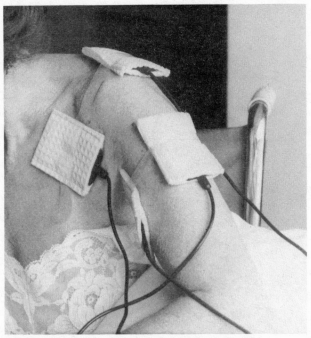

Fig. 8/2   Biceps tendinitis: arrangement of electrodes

It is interesting to note that with these patients a decrease of pain and an increased range of movement do not occur simultaneously. Some patients report that from the first few treatments although the pain is as severe as ever the shoulder moves more easily; another reports that although the pain is better and he is able to sleep on that side, the stiffness is as bad as ever. In all cases, the second disability begins to improve after an interval. It is found that exercise, particularly immediately after the interferential therapy, retards restoration of function. If the patient does no exercises the range of movement progressively increases, but the harder he tries the less satisfactory the result will be. Rest, with interferential therapy, will restore function.

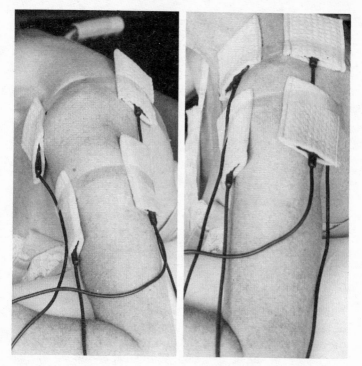

Fig. 8/3 Capsulitis of the glenohumeral joint: arrangement of electrodes

Fig. 8/4 Supraspinatus tendinitis: arrangement of electrodes

9. Treatment of Back Pain and Disc Lesions

Acute back pain is very effectively treated with interferential therapy. Treatment may be begun as soon as possible after onset, even if the patient is confined to bed or on traction.

When the pain is confined to the back, treatment is given exactly as for spondylosis (see p. 81), except that progress will be slower and either a constant sedative frequency or a very small sweep in the 90–130Hz range should be given for several days.

In-patient treatment

If the patient is in bed he must be disturbed as little as possible; he should be helped gently on to one side by an assistant while the operator places the electrodes under the back, two above and two below the site of the lesion. With a patient on leg traction this is relatively easy, but is more difficult, though still possible, for a patient on pelvic traction. The patient then rolls back in to lying thus holding the electrodes in place.

When the pain is referred down the leg, treatment to the spine is followed by treatment to the leg. Two electrodes are placed on the foot and the other two under the buttock so that the current traverses the whole length of the nerve. Sedative treatment (100 or 130Hz) or a small sweep, 90–100Hz, is given for 10 minutes.

Outpatient treatment

When the patient is no longer bedfast but is able to come to the department, he may be treated in any position he finds tolerable. If he does not wish to sit or lie, using vacuum electrodes he may even be treated in standing. He may be treated in lying, prone lying, side lying or sitting leaning forward on to a plinth. Treatment in lying has been described.

In side lying or prone lying vacuum electrodes are most convenient and comfortable (Fig. 9/1). In this position it is much easier to be sure of accurate siting. The site of the lesion can be found accurately by exploring with the glove electrodes as already described (see p. 47), and often tender places can be

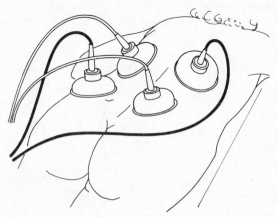

Fig. 9/1   Lumbago: treatment in prone lying using 4 vacuum electrodes

located of which the patient has been unaware. Treatment is given with a constant frequency sedative current for 10–15 minutes, at an intensity to cause no contraction.

It can often be seen before treatment that part of the erector spinae is in spasm, and the patient will certainly be aware of this. When the current has been flowing for some time the patient may report that the spasm has quite suddenly released, and this relaxation can sometimes be seen by an observer. Testing the area again with glove electrodes shows that the former hypersensitivity has disappeared. The spasm having been released, it is now possible to perform a manipulation if this is desirable. After manipulation, the patient often feels considerable pain over the site of the reduced disc. A three-times-toleration dose to this point allows the patient to leave the department free from pain. He must of course be given instructions as to which movements to avoid while the part is anaesthetised so as not to re-displace the disc.

If the trauma is not severe a single treatment may suffice, but usually a course of treatment is required. As soon as the pain and spasm are relieved after the sedative treatment, (and do not return before the next day) a sweep is gradually introduced to

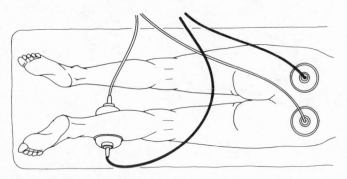

Fig. 9/2   Treatment of sciatica

increase the circulation and accelerate healing, and later to give gentle stimulation to the muscles.

If pain is referred down the leg the back treatment is followed by a longitudinal treatment with two electrodes over the lumbo-sacral roots and two below the lower limit of pain (Fig. 9/2). If the pain extends to the foot the electrodes are placed on the sole and dorsum. However, if the pain extends only to the calf the electrodes are placed on either side of the ankle, and if it is referred only to the ischial tuberosities the electrodes are placed on either side of the thigh. Usually as the back condition clears up the extent of the pain becomes less, so the position of the electrodes alters from treatment to treatment. Often the patient is left with severe residual pain in the ischial tuberosity, and a strong three-times-toleration dose to this area brings relief. It is clear that this dose is not being given to the site of the lesion causing the pain but probably influences the circulation to the point through the autonomic nerves.

Some patients with sciatica respond better to treatment with the two-electrode method. One electrode is placed on the affected disc and the other just below the lower limit of referred pain. The pattern of treatment is exactly the same as with the four-electrode method.

A course of 12 treatments beginning daily and becoming less frequent as the relief of pain lasts longer is usually sufficient. In long-standing cases, particularly those which have resisted other forms of treatment, it will take longer. After five days, frequency of treatment should be decreased to three times a week to avoid tiring the patient, but treatment may be continued for six to eight weeks if necessary, so long as some relief of pain is still obtained.

10. Treatment of Incontinence

Urinary incontinence is a most distressing and obstinate condition, but is amenable to interferential therapy in cases where there is a loss of sphincter control. Clearly it cannot be effective for all incontinent patients since many, particularly after childbirth, have gross structural damage which must first be repaired. Unfortunately it often happens that when surgical repair has been made, apparently satisfactorily, the patient remains incontinent due to sphincter weakness or faulty autonomic innervation. This can, however, be treated with interferential therapy with excellent results. It may not be successful in all cases of nocturnal enuresis in children, since there is often an underlying psychological disturbance which no electrical treatment could cure.

Successful results have been obtained in the treatment of all three types of incontinence: senile, stress and nocturnal enuresis. The success rate is encouraging, and since the treatment involves no discomfort or inconvenience to the patient it is worth trying in all cases.

Treatment aims at increasing the efficiency of the sphincter by stimulating the unstriped muscle with low frequency impulses to which it is sensitive and also by influencing the autonomic supply. This is more likely to succeed than the more usual methods of faradism and exercises which can only influence the sphincter indirectly through association with the striped muscle of the pelvic floor. Since it is desirable that the sphincter control is entirely unconscious, it must be treated through the involuntary muscle and the autonomic nervous system. Voluntary muscle of the pelvic floor is also in the path of the current and will receive its share of the treatment; therefore, teaching pelvic floor exercises will accelerate recovery. Nevertheless, this treatment is found to be effective even when the patient is unable or unwilling to do any voluntary exercises. Passage of current through the pelvic floor also accelerates repair of tissues damaged during delivery or at operation.

Treatment is given most conveniently using vacuum electrodes, but if these are not available plate electrodes may be used. It makes no difference to the efficiency of the treatment, only to the convenience of the operator.

Following childbirth, treatment may be initiated as soon as any difficulty is experienced. The condition might well be one that would right itself in time but it is unnecessary to allow it to persist if it can be cleared up quickly. Should the damage be more serious and require surgical repair, interferential treatment will increase local circulation and increase healing. No passive congestion is produced, so there is no danger of starting haemorrhage.

Treatment position

The patient is placed in stride sitting or crook stride lying. The elderly patient who comes to the department in a wheelchair need not be moved out of it as this position is ideal. Two electrodes are placed on the lower abdomen just above the outer half of the inguinal ligament. The medium size (10cm (4in)) vacuum cup is most suitable. The small cups are not so comfortable and, particularly with an elderly patient with a very fine skin, bruising may result. If plate electrodes are used they should be of similar size. The other two electrodes are placed on the upper part of the inner aspect of the thigh near the origin of the adductors (Fig. 10/1). These must be placed sufficiently far back to direct the currents through the pelvic floor with the crossing point at the urethral sphincter. Placing the electrodes too anteriorly will direct the current through the superficial tissues, missing the target entirely. If it is desired to treat the anal sphincter, which lies more posteriorly, the lower electrodes are placed more anteriorly and the upper moved from the abdomen to lie over the sacro-iliac joints. This produces a crossing in the posterior part of the pelvic floor.

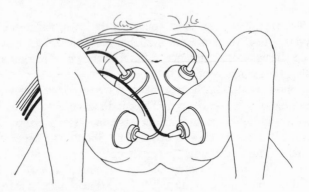

Fig. 10/1 Position of electrodes for treatment of incontinence. The patient is supported in crook stride lying

Treatment

A sweep of 0–100Hz is used. The lowest frequencies stimulate the unstriped muscle directly; 10–50Hz stimulate the voluntary muscles of the pelvic floor; and 5–100Hz the autonomic nerves. This can readily be appreciated by the normal subject who knows what to expect. It is helpful in explaining to the patient what she should feel if the operator has experienced the current herself.

The intensity of current is that required to produce a barely perceptible contraction of the pelvic floor, occurring only when the frequency is in the 10–50Hz range and followed by relaxation. The current must never be so strong as to produce a tetanic contraction lasting the whole cycle. The first treatment lasts eight minutes and the time is increased by one minute each attendance up to 15 minutes. The intensity of current is not increased; in fact as the condition of the muscle improves it is often found that less current is needed to produce the contraction.

Treatment is given two or three times a week. If it is given more frequently, it is too tiring for the patient and, in any case, time must be allowed for the muscle to become trained. Less frequently than twice a week is ineffective. A course of 12 treatments should be sufficient. With cases of recent onset the patient may be cured in fewer treatments, and it is not necessary to finish the course. Chronic, particularly senile, cases will need the full course and indeed may require a second course after an interval of two to four weeks. Patients usually report some slight improvement after two or three treatments even in cases of very long standing. Some senile patients cannot report progress and follow-up enquiries must be made with the nursing staff.

BRUISED PERINEUM

The same position of electrodes and the general procedure is followed for the treatment of a bruised perineum following childbirth. Not only is the condition acutely uncomfortable but, if the bruising is not rapidly resolved, lasting damage may be done to the pelvic floor. As there is pain a 10-minute constant 130Hz treatment is given, followed by a 10-minute sweep of 50–100Hz working up to 10–100Hz as quickly as possible to disperse the swelling.

The great advantage of this method is that no electrodes are placed on or near the perineum so reducing the likelihood of introducing infection or causing pain to the patient. The presence of clips or sutures presents no obstacle. The patient can wear normal protective clothing or a pad during treatment. Treatment is not uncomfortable and the slight contraction relieves the tension from the first treatment. Treatment is given daily until the bruising has gone, decreasing the time of sedative current and increasing the time of the sweep as the pain decreases.

The treatment may also be used in treating incontinence following prostatectomy and also for the relief of a non-specific prostatitis.

11. Treatment of Thoracic and Circulatory Conditions

ASTHMA

Treatment with interferential therapy will often give considerable relief to patients suffering from asthma. In this condition, expiration is impeded by spasm of the unstriped muscle of the bronchioles. The aim of treatment is to relax these muscles, enabling the lungs to collapse as the inspiratory muscles relax.

Treatment position

The patient is treated sitting in an upright chair. Two electrodes are placed on the back over the upper part of the trapezius and two anteriorly over the lower ribs (Fig. 11/1). If the patient is having difficulty in breathing while treatment is in progress he may find it more comfortable to sit leaning slightly forward with his arms supported on a table. In this case, the upper electrodes are placed anteriorly over the apices of the lungs and the lower electrodes posteriorly over the lower ribs. This position may also prove more convenient for a well-developed lady.

Treatment

A sweep of 10–100Hz is applied for 10 minutes at the first treatment, increasing by one or two minutes at each attendance up to a maximum of 20 minutes. Treatment is given three times a week for a month.

Because the heart is in the path of the current, this treatment should not be given to patients with a history of cardiac disease. All patients *must* be kept under close supervision during

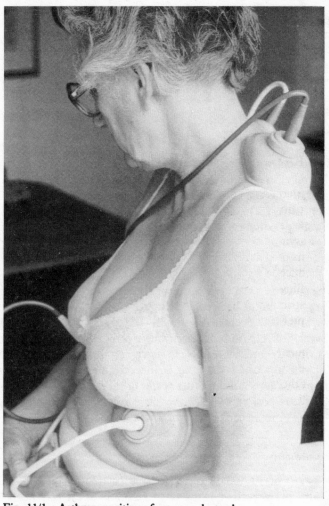

Fig. 11/1   Asthma: position of vacuum electrodes

treatment, and the current *must* be turned off at the least sign of distress.

During and after a course of treatment the breathing becomes progressively easier and the frequency of the acute attacks is reduced. A mild acute attack does not contra-indicate treatment since the patient is in no way restricted and indeed the relaxation induced will abort the attack.

TREATMENT OF CIRCULATORY DISORDERS

Interferential therapy is indicated in many cases of impaired circulation. Its action is directly through the stimulation of the muscular coats of the blood vessels and also by stimulation of the parasympathetic system. This is in contrast to the effect of most forms of electrotherapy which, by generating heat in the part, produce a passive congestion and so often an increase of swelling. Sympathetic stimulation would produce a vaso-constriction and is therefore contra-indicated. **Therefore the frequencies 0–5Hz must be avoided**. Using apparatus where this is impossible it must be borne in mind that in using frequencies 0–100Hz, 5 per cent of the cycle will be counter-productive.

If there is a history of thrombosis interferential must *never* be used on the affected limb. If a person has had a coronary thrombosis interferential must *not* be given.

To improve circulation

To increase the circulation of a leg two electrodes are placed one on either side of the lumbar spine; one on the dorsum and the other on the sole of the foot. A sweep of 10–100Hz is applied for 20–45 minutes at an intensity which produces a very gentle contraction in the *motor* part of the cycle only. A tetanic contraction of the voluntary muscle during the whole cycle is obviously contra-indicated, but the intermittent contraction of the muscles enhances the direct effect of the current on the blood vessels themselves.

Treatment is given three times a week for a month. For a condition such as *chronic chilblains* which recur year after year, treatment is best given in the autumn before the cold weather starts as a preventive measure and repeated if, or when, the chilblains appear. The treatment may have to be repeated for several years before the effect is permanent, but the condition becomes progressively less severe.

The same treatment is used for *chronically cold feet* and for *erythema nodosum*. If the condition has led to ulceration this is no contra-indication as the electrodes are placed above and below the ulcerated area without disturbing the dressing. The rate of healing is accelerated and the patient is much more comfortable. The type of dressing and frequency of renewal is a matter for discussion with the physician in charge of the patient, but need make no difference to the treatment.

Intermittent claudication

Treatment of intermittent claudication, while not entirely satisfactory, at least keeps the condition partially under control. It is not suggested that the patient is cured, but while he is having treatment the distance walked without pain increases and the foot remains warm with no sign of gangrene. On ceasing treatment unfortunately the patient slowly relapses. Treatment is given twice a week with two electrodes on either side of the calf just below the knee and two on either side of the ankle. A sweep of 10–100Hz is applied for 10 minutes initially, rising by two minutes each treatment to a maximum of 20 minutes. It may be necessary to continue the treatment indefinitely with suitable breaks for holidays, but other methods are no more satisfactory.

Lymphoedema

Patients with grossly swollen legs, either idiopathic or due to inactivity through being confined to a wheelchair or paralysed, are best treated with a sweep of 45–90Hz. This is because these frequencies have the greatest effect on the muscle coats of the blood vessels. It is obviously useless to try to obtain the assistance of the voluntary muscles if these are paralysed, so the lower frequencies which stimulate these are omitted. Treatment is given with the electrodes placed as before at an intensity to produce marked, but comfortable, prickling. Care must be taken not to give an overdose as the limiting feeling of 'tightening' will not be present in a paralysed limb. Treatment length starts at 20 minutes rising gradually to 45 minutes.

This treatment may also be given to a swollen arm following mastectomy. The current is not directed through the site of the primary cancer. The patient reports the limb as feeling lighter and more comfortable.

Sudeck's atrophy

Sudeck's atrophy is a resistant condition which responds well to interferential therapy, though treatment may have to be prolonged.

The four-electrode method is used. Two pads are placed on the forearm and the other two on the front and back of the hand. If available the largest size of combined electrode with pads of 5cm (2in) diameter may be used (if the arm is not too fat). A 100Hz constant or a sweep of 90–100Hz is applied at an intensity just short of contraction for 10 minutes working up to 15 minutes. Treatment is given three times a week for four to six weeks.

Both appearance and function of the hand begin to improve after a few attendances, but full recovery may take some time.

MIGRAINE

Many sufferers from migraine have reported that interferential therapy applied during an attack relieves the headache slowly, but more quickly than would be expected naturally. If available, a two-electrode method is used; one pad over the forehead and the other on the nape of the neck. A mild sedative treatment is given of 100 or 130Hz for 10–15 minutes. If applied in the *early* stage of an attack, it will be aborted.

A course of treatment two or three times a week for 12 treatments reduces both the frequency and severity of attacks.

12. Suggested Treatment Regimes

Ankle: sprained (see Figs. 5/1, 5/2)

1st treatment
Analgesic 15 minutes.
Local anaesthetising dose.
Strapping.

2nd treatment
Analgesic 15 minutes.
Strapping not removed.

3rd and subsequent treatments
Analgesic time gradually reduced.
Sweep gradually introduced; range and time progressively increased.

When the strapping is removed because it has become loose an anaesthetising dose is repeated, if necessary.

Asthma (see Fig. 11/1)

A sweep of 10–100Hz for 10 minutes, increasing to 15 minutes.

Calf muscle: torn fibres (see Figs. 5/3, 5/4)

1st treatment
Analgesic dose 15 minutes.
Local anaesthetising dose.
Strapping.

2nd treatment
Analgesic dose using the four-electrode method for 15 minutes.

3rd and subsequent treatments
Analgesic dose gradually reduced.
Small sweep introduced; range and time gradually increased.

Strapping should not be removed for three weeks if still effective.

Cervical spine (see Fig. 7/5)

Analgesic 7–15 minutes.
A sweep of 10–100Hz for 10–15 minutes.
Total treatment time 15 minutes.

Heberden's nodes (painful) (see Fig. 7/6)

Analgesic 7–10 minutes.

Hip: osteoarthritis (see Figs. 7/1, 7/2)

Treatment of hip joint
Analgesic 7 minutes.
Sweep of 10–100Hz 7 minutes.

Treatment of lumbar region
A sweep of 10–100Hz 7 minutes .

Impaired circulation of legs

A sweep of 10–100Hz for 15–45 minutes.

Intermittent claudication

A sweep of 10–100Hz for 15–30 minutes.

Knee

CRUCIATE LIGAMENT STRAIN

Timing and dosage as for lateral ligaments (see below).

MEDIAL LIGAMENT STRAIN (see Fig. 5/5)

1st treatment
Analgesic 15 minutes or longer if the swelling is gross.

2nd treatment
Analgesic 15–20 minutes.

3rd treatment
Analgesic dose gradually reduced.
Small sweep gradually increasing in range and size.

OSTEOARTHRITIS (see Figs. 7/3, 7/4)

Treatment of knee joint
Analgesic 7 minutes.
Sweep of 10–100Hz 7 minutes.

Treatment of lumbar region
Sweep of 10–100Hz 7 minutes.

Lumbago (see Fig. 9/1)

Acute phase
Analgesic 15–30 minutes.

Subacute phase
Analgesic 10–15 minutes. A small sweep gradually increasing in
range and duration to a total treatment time of 15–20 minutes.
When pain is localised, a three-times-toleration dose is given to
the tender area.

Post-herpetic neuralgia (see Figs. 6/1, 6/2, 6/3)

Intercostal nerve
(1) *Nerve roots*: Analgesic 10 minutes.
(2) *Nerve distribution*: Analgesic 10 minutes.

Trigeminal nerve
Mandibular, maxillary and frontal branches: Labile treatment 10–15 minutes to the affected branch(es).

Sciatica (see Fig. 9/2)

Acute phase
Analgesic 15–30 minutes.

Subacute phase
Analgesic 10–15 minutes.
A small sweep gradually increasing in range and duration as the analgesic dose decreases. As the extent of pain decreases the lower electrodes are moved up the leg.
When the pain is localised to the ischial tuberosity a three-times-toleration dose is given to this area.

Shoulder (see Figs. 8/1, 8/2, 8/3, 8/4)

Capsulitis; subdeltoid bursitis; supraspinatus tendinitis; biceps tendinitis.

Acute phase
Analgesic only for 15–20 minutes.

Subacute phase
Analgesic 7–15 minutes.
A small sweep of 5 minutes gradually increasing in range and duration. Total treatment time 15 minutes.
Cervical spine: A sweep of 10–100Hz for 5–7 minutes. When the pain is localised, give a three-times-toleration dose to the tender spot.

Sudeck's atrophy

A sweep of 90–100Hz for 7 minutes, gradually increasing to 15 minutes.

Temporomandibular joint (Fig. 12/1)

Analgesic 10–15 minutes.
A sweep for 5–7 minutes.
Total treatment time 15 minutes.

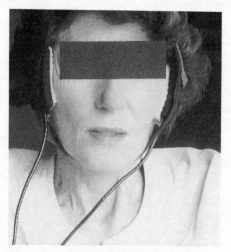

Fig. 12/1   OA temporomandibular joint:
arrangement of electrodes

Tennis elbow (see Figs. 5/6, 5/7, 5/8)

1st treatment
Analgesic; four-electrode method 15–20 minutes.
Local anaesthetising dose.

2nd treatment
Analgesic only, using the two-electrode method.

Tenosynovitis

1st-3rd treatments
Analgesic 10–15 minutes.

4th treatment
Analgesic 10 minutes.
A small sweep gradually increasing in range and duration to a total treatment time of 20 minutes.

Urinary incontinence (see Fig. 10/1)

A sweep of 10–100Hz for 7 minutes increasing gradually to 15 minutes.

Further Reading

Ganne, J. M. et al (1979). Interferential therapy to promote union of mandibular fractures. *Australian and New Zealand Journal of Surgery*, **49**, 1, 81–3.

McQuire, W. A. (1975). Electrotherapy and exercises for stress incontinence and urinary frequency. *Physiotherapy*, **61**, 10, 305–7.

Melzack, R. (1973). *The Puzzle of Pain: Revolution in Theory and Treatment*. Penguin Education Books, Harmondsworth.

Melzack, R. and Wall, P. D. (1982). *The Challenge of Pain*. Penguin Education Books, Harmondsworth.

Nikolova-Troeva, L. (1967). Interference-current therapy in distortions, contusions and luxations of the joints. *Münchener Medizinische Wochenschrift*, **109**, 11, 579–82.

Nikolova, N. (1969). Physiotherapeutic rehabilitation in the presence of fracture complications. *Münchener Medizinische Wochenschrift*, **111**, 11, 592–9.

Willie, C. D. (1969). Interferential therapy. *Physiotherapy*, **55**, 12, 503–5.

Index